She who brings life

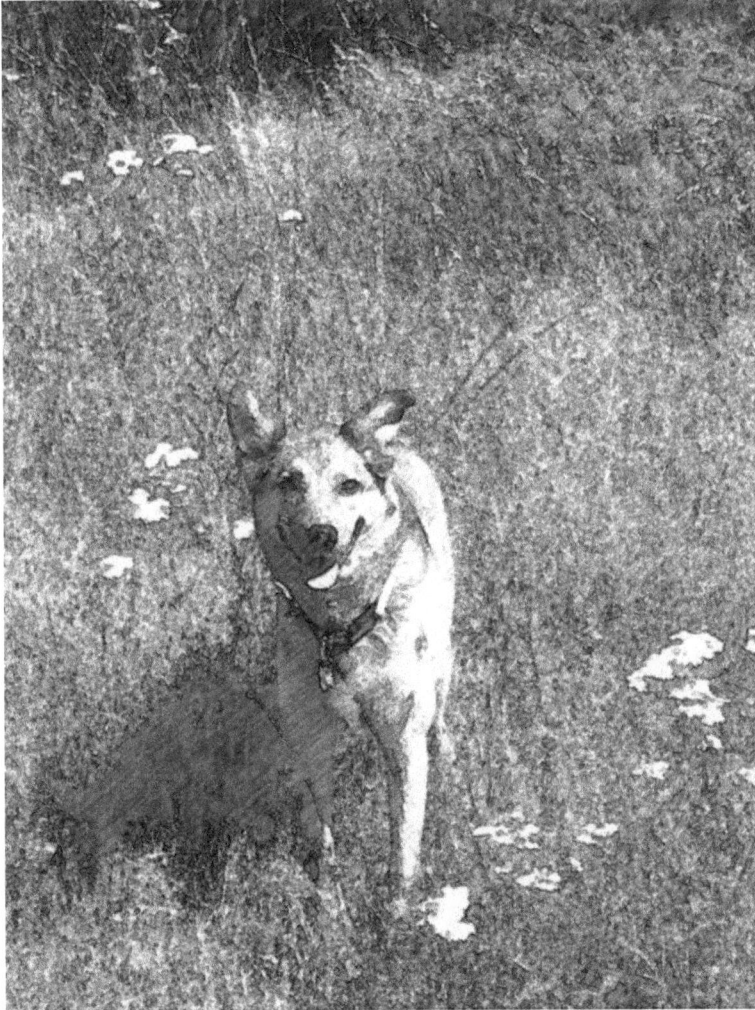

Michael Yanuck MD PhD

DEDICATION

In memory of Ini,
My soul dog,
2011-2023

And for Albert White Hat Sr., Phillip Whiteman Jr., Duane Hollow
Horn Bear, Nanette Antoine, Randy Jordan, Phillip Scott,
Kristine Turley, Sandy Swift Eagle, Mike Ryan,
Ruth & Curtis Thomas, Dan Foster,
Juan, Yanira & Carlos Rodriguez,
Joan Esnayra, Cinnamon Spear,
my wife,
and all the unnamed individuals of the Reservation
who took me into their lives and hearts and made this work possible.

.

The wilderness exemplifies the fullest potential of a life of exile: that the place where everything has been lost can prove to be the place where everything is gained.
~ David Damrosch

CHAPTER ONE

On a cold, subzero winter night in the Northern Plains, those inside the sweat lodge crawled out through the canvas flap into the elements. I was among the last to leave. The others, having formed a line, had already begun the ritual of shaking hands.

"Mitakuye Oyasin [We are all related]," we exchanged. "Mitakuye Oyasin."

Coming to tribal elder, Orville White Buffalo, he held my hand in both of his.

"Doctor, I'm sorry to hear about your wife," he said. "I prayed for her. I think we all did."

I nodded.

"Doctor, we're glad you're here," he continued. "We're glad you came back. I don't know the circumstances – I think it might not have been of your choosing – but I wanted you to know that I for one am glad your home."

The line dispersed. Crossing the jagged, frozen snow, I reached down to where my clothes lay. But instead of clothing, my hand encountered something small and naked, like an infant?!

Assuming it must be a wild animal, I sprang back, hoping whatever it was would do the same. But, to my surprise, it didn't, and instead emitted a chorus of sweet, sorrowful moans. Attempting to make out the identity of the creature, I narrowed my eyes. But there wasn't enough light. I looked to the heavens; it was a moonless night with an odd belt-like river of stars that stretched from one end of the horizon all the way to the other.

The Milky Way? I thought.

But even under the light of all the stars in the galaxy, the creature remained a mystery, shrouded in darkness.

Then, from the embers of the fire pit used to heat the ceremonial stones came a sudden 'crack', and the corresponding burst of light gave form to the creature.

It's a dog, I thought. A puppy.

I reached down and caressed its soft fur; but this seemed of little reassurance to the small animal, as it continued to whimper.

"Did someone lose a dog?" I called out. "There's a puppy here."

From around the ceremonial grounds sprang a chorus of good-natured naysaying.

"Not my dog, Dr. Mike," one said.

"Not my dog," said another.

"You better take that dog, Doc," said a third, "or else it's going to wind up in the soup."

In the general laughter that followed, I worked determinedly to extract my clothes out from under it.

With each article of clothing I removed, I expected the little thing to get to its feet and scurry off.

But it remained.

Finally, removing the last of my clothing, the animal fell back in the frozen snow, belly up, motionless and silent.

Rising to a stand, the little creature was swallowed up in the darkness created by the space between us. I gazed in the direction of the gate. The others had left and the grounds were silent.

I could leave, too, I thought. There was nothing to stop me – No one to tell me otherwise.

Then I thought, What about a little piece of joy for me in life? Why not? Why not a little piece of joy for me?

And acting on that spontaneous impulse, I bent low and wrapped the pup in my towel, then tucked it under my arm and whisked it away to my car; the pup offering no resistance, as its weight sank contentedly into my hand...

CHAPTER TWO

"Why did you take it?" my wife, April, asked when I called and told her about the puppy shortly after I got home.

How could I not? I responded. An innocent, little puppy with nowhere to go and no one to take care of it? I couldn't leave it.

Seated in the kitchen I watched the puppy roam the tile floor. It was my first real look at it. Still caked in snow, it had a beautiful coat of golden fur. Head up, bright and shiny, it pranced about the house without fear or apprehension.

"Like Socks," April said. "She needed us, too. Do you remember the day we found her before that storm? Can you hear her over the phone?"

Socks meowed in the background; I imagined April scooping her into her lap two thousand miles away at her grandmother's.

"Hmm, I wonder if the puppy will get along with cats?" she said. "Is it a he or a she?"

It's a she, I said. A sweet, little girl.

"Did you like it that she lied on your clothes?" she asked. "She was obviously cold. That's why she was on top of them. That and really smart: It knew the one thing that it could do, so you would take it home."

"Think about it," she continued. "Would you have taken it home if it'd jumped on you?... What if it had rubbed against your leg? Would you have brought it home then? If it had done anything else, you would have just brushed it aside, right? But, by lying on your clothes, it found the one thing that it could do to get you to take it with you. You wouldn't leave it lying there in the snow."

Yes, a desperate act of resignation. Such is what it takes to elicit some feeling from me.

April laughed. "She probably thought, 'I'm going to go to the Sweat Lodge and find myself a nice Jewish doctor. There's going to be one there.' Then, she sniffed you out. 'Those are the clothes of the Jewish guy. I'm going to plop myself down right here, and I'm not getting off until he takes me home. Do you have a name for her?"

Inipi, I said. The Lakota word for the Sweat Lodge ceremony, where she chose me.

"Hmmm," she responded. "You might want to change that. I don't know how the people there would take to you naming your dog after one of their ceremonies. Why don't you call her, 'Ini'?"

Okay, Ini it is...

The general store having long since closed, I fed Ini some leftovers from the casino.

In the bedroom I laid a pile of clothes for her to sleep on. But Ini circled the bed, calling out in sweet, sorrowful barks, until finally I lifted her in with me. There, she settled at the foot of the bed and curled into a ball and went to sleep.

At three in the morning, though, I awoke to the sensation of tiny creatures jumping all over me.

Fleas! I thought.

Lifting Ini from her place of peaceful slumbers, I deposited her on the back porch. Outside, more than barked, Ini howled, and listening I couldn't be sure whether it was for lost freedom, or loneliness? Whether I'd brought home a dog, or a little wolf?...

CHAPTER THREE

In the morning I woke to the sunrise, and went to the door to let Ini in. But Ini was nowhere to be found, and inspecting the yard, I discovered a hole in the fence.

She must have slipped through, I thought.

Going to the front porch, I called her.

"Ini... Ini..."

Nothing stirred.

I experienced a sinking feeling in my chest. It seemed my association with the sweet creature was meant to be a short one, I thought. That little pup really filled my heart.

Then, in the distance, came the sound of a faint yapping. Looking into the rising sun I saw a faint silhouette in the direction of the sound. As the figure grew nearer, I made out a large dog at his side – and something else that looked like a tiny, hopping dot?

As the three approached the house, I recognized my neighbor, Ryan (the hospital's health educator), jogging with his Siberian husky, Bright Eyes, and trailed by Ini.

"Yeah, the pup joined us not long after we started from the house," Ryan said. "I didn't think that the pup would keep up, but she ran with us the full three miles."

Ini wagged her whole body as she scurried around me...

CHAPTER FOUR

"I think you ought to call her, 'Walks Happy'," Ryan continued, "because of the way she's always wagging every part of herself. Do you have a name for her?"

I said my wife and I picked the name Ini for her, and apologized for her howling last night.

"Oh, she's got fleas?" he responded. "I got something for you, Doc. Follow me."

He led me to his garage.

"Now where did I put it?" he said. "Oh, here it is."

He brought out a flea collar.

"It might be a little big," he said. "Bright Eyes is quite a bit bigger than Ini... Do you know how Ini got out? I can help you look for a break in the fence that Ini might have slipped through. I'm pretty handy at that sort of thing. I used to live in your house before I took this one."

After sealing the fence Ryan and I set off on the short walk to the hospital.

"So, how are you liking it out here, Doc?" he asked.

I live and breathe for the kind of medicine I get to practice here, I said. Treatment that makes sense; doing the most with the least; attending the most vulnerable.

I love the nature; the vast open plains; the blankets of snow that eclipse all the constructs of man from view. Sometimes, I want to get lost in it. Others, the remoteness of the Reservation gets to me, and the isolation feels too much.

"I understand how you feel, Doc," he responded. "I know what it is to come from another world. You see, I was one of those Native American children who was adopted at birth. When that happened, I was removed from the Reservation and sent off to St. Paul. I wound up in the loving care of two very beautiful and loving parents. I had the best of memories as a little boy. But one strange twist was that I was never told that I was a Native American child. It was still taboo back then to openly proclaim that you had Native American descent or lineage in your family tree. And so, many times, it was kept secret, or even worse just swept under the rug."

"I was told that I was adopted," he continued. "But I was given the explanation that I was French Canadian. Well, that was partially correct – one quarter correct when you left out the Lakota part.

"The years went by, and then I lost both my adopted parents in a car crash. And it was my wife who, while gathering their belonging, stumbled upon my adoption papers.

"She kept the information secret from me; then, a few months later, I received a phone call, and there on the other end of the line was a gentleman who introduced himself as my biological brother. My wife had discovered him; neither of us had known of the others existence for all those years. His first words to me were, 'Hey, bro, you are Lakota.'

"We went on to exchange our life stories; but it was what he said at the conclusion of that call that was forever to change our destiny for my family and me, when he simply said, 'Come home. Com'on home.'

"We did. With the faith of my wife, we packed up all that we had, living in a comfortable suburb of Minneapolis, and headed west, to this Sioux Reservation. And here we were given a king's welcome. In the blink of an eye we were made to feel like part of the family, part of the community, part of the tribe, and part of this brand new world.

"I truly feel the product of two worlds – native America and mainstream America. And these are two worlds and two cultures who had been at odds with each other over and throughout the time of America's growing pains. You have to come to a point where you can embrace those two worlds and find the best in both.

"I am a son of two mothers, with a pride and respect for both. And it is there - from that place in between - that I do my work and serve the people every day. It's what I like to call 'reconciliation' – working for peace, hope and unity.

"You see, for the Lakota, our lives are about a journey that inevitably forms a circle in which there is no beginning and no end. The honoring of the circular nature of our lives as human beings is very important to us. If there's one message that I'd like to leave with you, it's that all of us – regardless of the color of our skin, or our religious backgrounds, or our political persuasions – we are simply human beings - brother and sisters of one heart, one mind, one body - in journey and quest and service of our Creator. I hope that the experience of being here will give that to you..."

CHAPTER FIVE

At the hospital clinic a patient with a knee injury returned for follow-up.

"The medicines you gave me are helping," he said. "I still feel pain there, but the swelling has gone down. I've gone back to walking. Maybe not the seven miles a day that I did before, but enough to go between people's houses."

"I've been through a lot worse than this, Doc," he confided. "Twenty years ago I was hit by a bus in Minneapolis. I was in the coma for weeks. I was kept alive by all kinds of machines. There were tubes down my throat that breathed for me, fed me. The doctors told my mother I wasn't gonna make it, and said she should let them turn off the machines that were keeping me alive. Even if I came out of it and I wasn't a vegetable, they said, I'd never do the things I used to. My mother said, 'He's too ornery to die. He's not ready yet.'

"She and my aunt sat with me. They brought a Medicine man from the Reservation to make ceremony and pray over me – for three and a half weeks, until I woke up.

"I had to re-learn everything. I had to learn how to walk. How to talk. It was like I didn't remember how to do anything. But my mother wouldn't let me quit. Every day I got a little stronger.

"The first time they got me up to walk, I stood up between those parallel bar, and fell right on my face. But before that, I took two steps!

"I lifted my hand to my doctors and put up two fingers. 'Okay,' they said. 'We see you. Yeah, two steps.' But I kept on holding up those two fingers – to let them know. That I wasn't a vegetable, and I was going to walk again, and I was going to talk, and they weren't right about me.

9

"It was still hard. Before the accident, I was really athletic. I could run faster than anyone. I could swim like a fish.

"When I got out of the hospital, I told them to take me to the top of the hill and I performed a VisionQuest. I asked *Tunkashila* why I was still here? Why he let me live? Why he didn't take me?

"And you know what I learned after those four days of being up there with nothing to eat or drink?... It was so I could tell others what had happened to me; and if I could do it – if I could get better - then they could, too.

"The world is too beautiful to just give up on it. That's what the experience taught me. That's what I learned..."

CHAPTER SIX

Returning home Ini wasn't in the yard. Despite reinforcing the fence, Ini must have found a way through again. As I walked the streets looking for her, a pickup truck slowed and pulled next to me.

"Are you lost, Doc?"

It was Ryan. When I told him Ini got out again, he drove ahead, saying he, too, would look for her. Within a few minutes, he was back.

"I found a mom and three puppies that look like Ini," he said. "These pups are about the same size and shape as Ini. It could be Ini's mom and siblings."

He brought me to a dilapidated house at the edge of the neighborhood; a mother dog and her pups were on the porch; except for darker fur, the pups were near identical to Ini.

"Should we knock on the door and ask if we can have one?" Ryan asked.

The young dogs appeared forlorn, and none exhibited the spark that Ini did; none approached or showed interest, and all seemed attached to their mother.

I think I'll keep looking, I told Ryan.

Ryan nodded, his gaze directed downward.

"I understand, Doc," he said. "Hope Ini comes home soon."

He went back to his truck, then turned.

"You heard in Morning Report about that stray dog with rabies that bit a little girl?" he said. "Well, the tribal police have been rounding up all the strays. The ones that try to get away, they just shoot. I'm not sure the ones they gather fare much better."

"Yeah," he concluded. "I sure do hope you find her..."

CHAPTER SEVEN

During the night I lay on the couch with the door open, hoping that Ini would wander in.

What is happening? I thought. When our cat, Socks, disappeared for a day, I shed no tears. Why were my feelings so different about this animal?

"Yeah, you're definitely attached to her," April said. "I wish I was there to help you look for her. I hope she turns up soon."

I could hear Socks in the background.

"She's okay," she said. "Actually, I took her to the vet because she's been getting thinner. The vet checked her out and gave her some stomach medicine. He didn't think it was anything serious. I think it's because she's missing you."

Listening, I recalled my last day with Socks before leaving. April was away receiving treatment, and I was packing my things when Socks did something I'd never seen her do before; she crawled into our bed and lay there, unmoving. Socks never went on the bed; the only place she ever slept or rested was her cat tower. I was so taken aback by her stillness that I observed her to make sure she was still breathing. Assured that she was alright, it struck me that it was as though she'd 'taken to bed.' Depressed. *Catatonic.*

Perhaps, my packing had rekindled a memory of what happened with her previous owner? And being deserted as a kitten, before April and I found her? Maybe, she was re-living that abandonment? Just a few months old, and no one to care for her.

I got into bed, and lay beside her. It will be alright, Socks. We'll be together again soon. You don't have to worry. I'll come back to you and April. It won't be long.

Then, my thoughts drifted to April, and I experienced a deep ache in my chest.

Wow, I thought, sitting back in the chair and breathing through the discomfort. How had I been there for Socks, and not April?...

CHAPTER EIGHT

Around noon I remembered that Orville had invited me for
another 'sweat.' I hurried to his home, but arrived as the ceremony
was ending.

"Hi Doctor," Orville said. "You weren't able to make it?"

I apologized, saying I'd lost the puppy and spent the morning
searching for her. He laughed.

"Don't worry, Doctor," he said. "That dog will find its way back
home again."

He sat heavily on a bench, and put on his clothes.

"Sometimes we feel down – mentally, physically," he said,
reassuringly. "We're down because we have too many problems,
frustrations – those things can really hold you down. And you go into
a sweat lodge and you deal with them. It seems to bring that life
back. These last few months I've really had a hard time with my
wind. They put me on chemo and I think they almost killed me. I
couldn't breathe. I was dizzy. They finally took me off that because
my cancer had spread. They put me on another pill and my wind is
shortly coming back. The interesting thing is – all the time I've
been having problems breathing, I'd go into a sweat lodge, and I'd
feel good. I'd breath good again. One time my daughter was in there
with us and she said, 'For somebody who couldn't breathe, you
couldn't stop singing in there.'"

He laughed.

"I kept singing because it felt good," he continued. "It's just
very interesting that inside there I could really breath good and
sing."

Getting up, he motioned me to follow.

14

"Com' on, doctor," he said. "We're gonna go in the house and have something to eat. Come and join us…"

In the dining room we gathered around the table, and recited a Lakota prayer song before the meal.

Du way waka-ta waka, Cha che waki ey lo hi.
Ti wa hey ki, Dy ya namach hu we lo hey yo.

The meal began with bowls of the buffalo stew passed around the table.

"Do you know what that song means, Doctor?" Orville asked.

For all that is sacred, I drum and sing.
For all of creation, I am grateful.

. "What is 'sacred', doctor?" he asked.

I suppose everything is sacred, I responded.

"In our way, *waka* – what you call sacred – to us is energy," he said. "It is the energy that can give or take life. Energy that can be used for creation or destruction. Good and evil are within this energy, and both are equally powerful."

Nodding, I thought of Ini.

"Do you know what 'Ini' means?" he asked.

I shook my head.

Just short for *Inipi,* I responded, where she chose me.

He sat quiet.

"*Ni* is 'he or she is alive'," he said. "That's what *Ni* means. *I* refers to the source that gives him or her life. *Inipi* really means is 'a place to bring life.'"

He leaned back.

"There's a story," he began, "about four brothers who lived together. One day this woman came to their lodge. She said, 'I've come to help you. I understand you're living by yourselves. So I've come to help you live.' So the brothers talked, and they took her in as a sister. They provided everything she needed. For them she made clothing. She cooked for them. And she provided for them all they needed.

"Then, one day, the oldest brother went out and never returned. And when he didn't come home for several days, the next one went looking for him. He never returned. Then, the third one. She begged the youngest not to go. And he said, 'That's my responsibility. It's my responsibility to find my brothers.' So she made him provisions and he left – he never returned, either.

"So one day she sat on this long hill, remembering her brothers. She was crying. She found this little pebble – It was perfectly round. She put it in her mouth. Then, she swallowed it by mistake. And that pebble made her pregnant. She had a boy that grew very fast into a man. And they lived and he provided.

"One day he said, 'What happened to your brothers?' So she told him what happened that day – That the one went out and never returned and the others went looking for him and they never returned. So he said, 'Make provisions for me. I'm going to find them.' She begged him not to go, and he said, 'That's the reason I came - to find my uncles.'

"So, she made provisions for him and said, 'They went in this direction.' So, he went in that direction and walked for a long time. He finally came to a tree. So he rested at that tree. And at that time we talked to other beings. With the birds. The four-legged. We communicated with them.

"So, while he was resting, this bird said, 'Keep going in this direction.' So, he rested and then he went and followed that direction. He went for a long time and then he came to a tree and he sat down to rest. And again the birds said, 'Yes, they came here. And then they went to that mountain. When you get to that mountain, a wuchasa – a man - will be waiting for you. Follow his directions very carefully.'

"So he went to that mountain and a *wicasa* – a man – was waiting for him. 'Go up to the top,' he said. 'When you get to the top, be very careful because this old woman is going to greet you. Be careful. And when you finish with her, there are some bundles in her lodge.' Then, he told him how to build a sweat lodge. He said, 'Build a structure, cover it, and then bring those bundles inside. Those four. And heat the stones – ten of them – and bring them in. And then pour water on the stones. But be very careful.'

"When he got to the top of the mountain, this little old lady greeted him. Said, 'Tokala. Go inside. I've been waiting for you. And I've prepared some stew for you – soup. You must eat.' So they went into her lodge. When they went in, he noticed those bundles in her lodge. He was going to sit down and this little old lady says, 'Grandson, before you sit down to eat, could you walk on my back. I have this back problem and when somebody walks on it, I feel so good.' She laid down on her stomach and he was looking down at her back and right along her spine, he could see some things kind of protruding against her dress – like sharp things were kind of pushing her dress up right along her spine. He stood there and watched her and finally he turned himself into a huge boulder – great big boulder – rock – and just rolled over – crushed her.

"After, he went back to himself and built that lodge – that Inipi lodge - just like this one." He motioned outside to his lodge. "And he heated the ten stones. When the stones were ready, he brought those four bundles in. He brought the stones in, covered it, covered the door and he poured water on the stones. And pretty soon, those bundles moved around. They said, 'Let us out.' So he opened the bundles, and his uncles came back to life."

"*Ni,*" he concluded. "*Ini. He or she who brings back life again...*"

CHAPTER NINE

The buffalo meat in the stew was tender.

"I always enjoy your authentic Lakota cooking," I told Orville. "I wish I could bring something authentic to my 'tribe', but I think all that was lost two thousand years ago with the destruction of the Temple."

"Well, Doctor, why not the next time you come, you bring some bagels and lox," he said. "I had that when I visited some Jewish people in Los Angeles, and it was really good. At first when they started saying stuff about 'lox', I thought they were talking about 'padlocks' to hold down the food. But when they brought it out, and I got to try it, I really liked it.

"I met them because I helped the patriarch of the family on the street. He was in dire need at the time; afterward, he called me 'a real mensch.' When I said I didn't know what that means, he told me it was Yiddish for a person of integrity and honor.

"He invited me to his home to meet his family. After that I broke many a matzo ball with them."

He laughed, then looked anxiously over his shoulder.

"Dr. Mike, before you go, can you please take a look at my daughter, Somay?" he said. "Her leg is all swollen."

He led me to the living room where a young woman wearing shorts and hiking boots was standing. And though I'd never seen her before, I felt an odd familiarity?

"Somay, I want the doctor to take a look at you," Orville said. "Show him your leg."

The young woman complied: Taking a seat on the couch, she pulled down her sock. Then, before I could kneel to examine the wound, she lifted the affected leg over her head.

18

Whoa! I thought, taken aback.

I wondered if this was some 'learned behavior'?... Obediently exposing oneself when confronted by someone of the medical professional?

Meanwhile, behind the calf was large, circular area of redness and swelling with a puncture mark in the center.

"Do you remember getting bit by something?" I asked.

"Well, I was opening the door to the attic, and this spider dropped on me," she said. "I remember it having a small body and really long legs."

Hmmm, I thought. Very observant.

"Probably a brown recluse," I responded. "Keep the area iced. That keeps the poison from working and gives the body time to degrade the venom. If it isn't considerably better by tomorrow, come to the clinic and we'll see about treating you with antibiotics."

"Thank you, Doctor," Orville interjected.

Then, as he led me back to the table, I received a text from Ryan.

Dr. Mike, Ini came back today. I put her in your garage. She's locked in.

"It's a sign," Orville said. "Ini found you at a Sweat. Now, she's been found right after another one..."

I excused myself and made a bee-line for home.

Opening the garage Ini greeted me; more than her tail, she wagged her whole body...

CHAPTER TEN

The house didn't have a washer and dryer, so I made a weekly trip to the laundromat at Wannapuk (the town bordering the Reservation) thirty miles south. While the wash was going, I led Ini into the nearby fields. But within a few yards, I found myself walking alone. Retracing my steps, I found Ini stopped and sitting. I tried to coax her, but she wouldn't come. There was no change in her expression; no look of pain, or barking, or whimpering; nothing to indicate anything out of the ordinary; she was just stopped and looking at me.

"What's the matter, Ini?"

I knelt and examined her and found her paws were full of barbs. From experience I knew these barbs were intensely sharp, but fortunately dissolved with the slightest application of moisture.

As I sat extracting the barbs, my thoughts drifted to an old girlfriend and her children. The children were given a bunny at an Easter festival, but, sadly, the animal had died within a week. This surprised me, as the animal didn't seem unwell? Inspecting the cage, I discovered the nozzle of the water dispenser didn't work reliably, and I surmised the animal had died of dehydration despite a full bottle of water right beside it.

What had this little creature been thinking? I wondered. It had never complained; never indicated any sign of distress. Just sat there staring up (with what seemed like an accusatory expression now), as though resigned to some assumed malevolent intent on our part?

Sitting now with Ini, I cradled her in my arms.

"I   hope   you   don't   feel   that   way,"   I   said...

20

CHAPTER ELEVEN

How could we actually take something that could kill us and it becomes our best friend and lives close with us, sleeping on our beds, but in the wild these are aggressive animals that routinely take down prey larger than themselves. So that, I think it is a wonderful puzzle.
~ Robert Wayne, biologist, University of California, Los Angeles

As the weeks past, life settled into a predictable routine. On Saturday mornings I went into town for coffee and to buy Ini a fifty-cent stuffed animal at the church-sponsored thrift store. Entering the thrift store this week, my eyes gravitated to a jigsaw puzzle in the window display, the pieces coming together to produce a puppy whose expression and coloring was not unlike Ini's. I was reminded of the puzzles April used to put together while I was away looking for jobs. Of late, she'd asked for a picture of Ini; but Ini was always in such constant motion that all I'd been able to achieve in photographs was a little blond blur!

"So you like puzzles!" the clerk said at the checkout counter. "When I was a little girl I used to love doing puzzles. I'd do the simple puzzles, like this one here. I'd do them over and over. Then, my mother insisted that I do more 'age appropriate' puzzles. I found them really difficult and frustrating and they lost all enjoyment for me. So, I stopped doing them."

I smiled.

"When I was maybe twelve," I commented, "I received some money from my grandparents for my birthday. When my mom asked what I wanted to do with the money, I said I wanted a mechanical toy dog."

I shook my head.

"Can you imagine?" I said. "What 12-year-old boy wants a mechanical toy dog for his birthday?"

"Did you have a dog?" she asked.

I shook my head.

No, I responded.

Then, it occurred to me I had? His name was Blackie – probably a black Labrador-German shepherd mix. He was just a puppy when my mom brought him home in a paper sack. She got him from a friend who found him wandering the condominium complex. I could still remember how he looked that night: Sweet, embarrassed, nervous, scared. From the start, he was my dog.

And that dog could do anything: Play soccor, frisbee, fetch. The only time he ever whined was when his neck got caught in the tetherball rope – My father was still with us then, because I remember it was he who went outside and untangled Blackie.

After my parents divorced, we moved to another house. The house didn't have a fenced-in backyard. I guess my mom hadn't thought about it before settling on the place. She didn't know how to do a lot of things. I guess she kind of relied on my dad for that. We chained the dog to a tree. I don't think Blackie liked that. He kept on getting tangled in the chain – wrapping it around and around the tree till he wound up stuck there.

And there was this small dog named Foxie. It belonged to our next-door neighbor. They would let it run free and it would come around into our backyard. I don't think it meant to tease Blackie – maybe, it did.

One night Blackie broke the chain and went after Foxie. It was just my younger brother and me that night (I don't know where my mother was). I went after Blackie and caught her across the street. I was pulling Blackie back to the house when he lounged and broke free. This time, he bit Foxie and shook her, tearing the skin. I grabbed Blackie, and my brother took Foxie. I'll never forget the sight of my brother's shirt, full of blood.

When my mom got home, we took Foxie to the vet and got her sewed up.

Returning to the house, my mother made some calls. Afterwards, she told me that Blackie had to go to the pound and we couldn't keep him anymore.

Blackie was locked in the bathroom. I went inside and stayed with him through the night. He was as gentle as he'd ever been. Nothing to be afraid of. Looking the same as he did when he was a puppy. Embarrassed. Scared.

The following day I went to school and spent the whole time crying. Classmates came by and asked, What's the matter? But when I told them, they didn't understand...

"So, you wanted a mechanical dog," the clerk reasoned, "that no one could ever take away."

Smiling, I nodded approvingly – She'd solved the puzzle!

"Do you have a dog now?" she inquired.

Yes, I said. Her name is Ini...

CHAPTER TWELVE

Arriving home Ini dipped her nose into the bags from the thrift store.

"Is there a gift for me?" she seemed to ask. "Where is my new toy?"

Then, locating the new stuffed animal I'd bought for her, it was time for her favorite game – Keep Away! The stuffed animal in her mouth, she positioned herself behind a tree, and dared me to take the toy from her. Then, just as I got close, she zipped away to the bush on the other side of the yard, with a speed and agility that was amazing to behold!

Even when I got close, she'd just get down low and accelerate beyond my reach. And looking on I wondered that native warriors had displayed similar feats on horseback to the awe of members of the Cavalry?

Then, running through some brush, charcoal-colored markings were left across her face.

Now you really look like an Indian brave, I thought. Wearing war paint.

My thoughts drifted to Frank Lightning, the Cheyenne healer who taught the children native horsemanship during my first stay here.

"If you're really interested in learning these ways," he'd told me, *"you'll come and see me in Montana..."*

It was only a year ago, but events in between made it seem like a lifetime...

At midday we drove out into the open plains beyond the medical complex; eagles soared overhead, and the chirping of frogs and insects created a cacophony of sound like a veritable symphony, and in this seemingly endless expanse of fields and wide open spaces, vast skies and other creatures, I felt at one with nature, and less insignificant.

In a field of flowers Ini sprang into the air, hopping and soaring after butterflies, as though to touch them with the tip of her nose. It was an amazing feat to watch – She looked just like a kangaroo!

Then, a shot rang out, and a patch of dirt kicked up not far from Ini, who stopped and looked back at me. From behind I heard the sound of galloping. Turning, I expected to see a horse; instead, it was a large brown hound, charging right at me. I raised my hands and stood solidly in the animal's path.

"No, no, no!" I shouted.

But it wouldn't veer and knocked me to the ground as it kept charging after Ini. Ini tried to outrun it, but the larger dog pounced and tackled Ini, sending her tumbling to the ground. Coming out of the roll, Ini yelped inconsolably – barking, barking, barking, like I'd never seen or heard her before. I ran to her.

"Ini, what's the matter?"

She just kept yelping, as though in some horrified state of shock!

Was the barking meant to ward off the bigger dog? I thought.

And there was something else, as well – Ini was 'sitting' as though anchored to the ground!

The large dog knelt nearby; positioned in the posture of the sphinx, its bearing suggesting recognition of some gravity of the event that was as yet unknown to me.

A man wearing camouflage gear approached. A rifle slung over his shoulder, he moved in slow, measured, self-assured steps.

"I saw that wild coyot' and thought I better shoot it," he said.

'Coyot'?!' I repeated. That's no coyote. 'That's my dog.

Ini kept yelping and wouldn't - or couldn't! – move from the spot she'd gone down. What's wrong with her? I thought. Why is she so plastered there? Is her back broken? The hunter looked on, unmoved.

"Sure is built like a coyot'," he said. "Bet she's a coy-dog. That's when a bitch is tied down and bred with coyotes. The offspring are used as decoys to draw the coyot's out, so hunters can shoot them."

Shaking my head I decided there was nothing to do but carry Ini back to the car and go for help. Lifting her, she let out a high pitched yelp and reflexively bit my nose. Then, looking into her panic-stricken eyes, I experienced something odd: a moment of tunnel vision, where Ini's terrified expression was all I could see.

"How did you get that dog?" the hunter asked.

"She chose me," I said. "At a Sweat Lodge ceremony."

25

"Oh, then she's a rescue," he said.

"Yeah," I said. "She rescued me..."

CHAPTER THIRTEEN

Ini couldn't have weighed more than forty pounds; but my arms were tiring even after a few hundred yards, as I struggled to carry her. Ini trembled as I searched for a place to put her down. On lowering her, Ini reacted by scampering away on three legs - the fourth (her hind left) dangling in an unnatural way. Looking on, I had my answer: It wasn't her back – It was her leg that was broken.

Ini crawled under a brush and lay panting, frothing at the mouth with her eyes rolled back in her head. For the first time since bringing her home, she was motionless; her tail didn't wag; there was no outward recognition of her surroundings. This animal for whom my every attempt to capture her on film had only produced a gold-brown blur, now showed no excitement, no hint of expression; only some inescapable resignation to the cruel fate events had dealt her; a death sentence meted out by nature that, however unfair, given the agony of her present condition, she did willingly accept.

I got under the brush and lay next to her, reassuringly stroking her fur.

"It will be alright, Ini," I said. "You'll be alright."

But Ini remained detached, breathing through what I could only imagine was immeasurable pain.

Perhaps, she thinks, 'This is it. I'm food for the wolves now.'

I looked out. What's left of life when you're without a leg to stand on? Here in this place of exile – this wilderness, this desert – from which there's no going back. No returning. No second chance.

Ini stopped hyperventilating, but appeared hardly conscious.

Such a lovely creature, I thought. Is this how it ends?...

CHAPTER FOURTEEN

Lifting Ini, I began to walk again; she offered no resistance this time, and I couldn't be sure it was because she'd given up or lost consciousness? The path was filled with flowers; some large and bright yellow; others white like poppies; and thistles of every imaginable purple hue. There were ferns and sprouting conifers. The fruit sprang from the succulents looked like dried bitter melon, reminiscent of the Asian farms I'd seen in DC. As we moved into a deep ravine, scattered sage filled the fields.

But the road was nowhere to be found.

"Ini, I'm sorry," I said. "I must have taken a wrong turn. I don't know where we are."

My arms were getting heavy again, and the trail was going on with no end. How can it be that one wrong turn has got us so miserably lost? How did these people do it? How could they possibly have carried their women and children between these distances – without the promise of food or water? Chasing the buffalo? How did they do it? Got to get us back to the road, and hope someone helps us.

It seemed every manner of thorn and burr lodged in my shoes, and ached with every step. I thought of the barbs in Ini's paws some weeks ago, so that she couldn't move anymore. How she hadn't whimpered. Had offered no sound. I thought about stopping; but I couldn't stop now; couldn't put Ini down again; not like this.

I began to wonder if this trail would ever get to the road, or just meander through the Reservation like the river?

I should have asked the hunter for help, I thought. But I was too proud. Too offended – Because of his lack of compassion. Lack of feeling. Lack of apparent concern. So I went off – now probably a

28

hundred times worse off than I would have been had I just asked for his assistance. Had I just turned back when I'd begun to suspect I didn't know where I was.

Finally, I found the road, but wasn't sure where the car was?

Won't someone help us? I thought. Someone please help us!

Just then, a beat-up, old station wagon slowed and pulled alongside us, the driver rolling down the window.

"Doctor, are you alright?"

It was a young woman I didn't recognize.

"It's my dog," I said. "I think she broke her leg."

"There's a pet hospital in town," she said. "I can take you if you like."

She opened the hatch; I laid Ini inside, still straining to recall where I knew her from?

"It's Somay," she said. "Orville's daughter. Dad asked you to look at my leg. You probably didn't recognize me because I changed my hair..."

She drove me to my car, then I followed her and Ini into town. The veterinary clinic was located just beyond the town square. Parking, I went to retrieve Ini. To my surprise, Ini wasn't in the back of the wagon, but just behind Somay.

"Ini stayed quiet for a while after you left," she said. "Then, suddenly, I was hearing yelps of pain. So, I looked over, and she was hobbling on three legs. I couldn't do anything because I was driving. And she walked from the back all the way to the front. And then she put her paws so they were on the edge of the backseat – to be as close to me as she can. And it was like the sweetest thing. Like she tolerated pain in order to get as close to me as she could. Then, she sat there. She's so sweet."

She stroked Ini's fur.

"Sweet girl," she said. "Sweet girl..."

CHAPTER FIFTEEN

The veterinarian assistant brought us into an examination room. Laying Ini on the stainless steel examination table, the assistant poked and prodded Ini. In between yelps of pain, Ini licked the assistant.

"Hmmm?" the assistant murmured. "What a sweet dog."

The assistant took Ini for X-rays, then brought her back a few minutes later.

"The veterinarian will come to talk with you after he's looked at the X-ray," the assistance said.

Smiling, Ini appeared her usual engaged and happy self. Still, the image of her laying in the brush (as though ready to accept death) kept flickering in my head.

"The way she looked," I confided to Somay. "It was like she'd given up on life."

"But you didn't give up on her, Dr. Mike," Somay responded.

Just then, a gangly fellow entered the room and slapped an X-ray film on the mounted light box on the wall.

"Your dog's leg is broken," he announced. "We'll need to put a pin in."

In the X-ray Ini's leg looked like a wishbone snapped in two.

"No running around for a while," the veterinarian continued.

The veterinarian turned his attention to Ini, examining her leg.

"You're pretty lucky you caught me," he said. "I was just about to go hunting. It's pheasant season. Best pheasant hunting in the country right here. You hunt?"

No, I responded, adding that there were mostly sage grouse where we were, and I hadn't seen many pheasants.

"I think the pheasants were brought over from China," he commented.

Then, he looked at us, grinning.

"But I guess that's okay," he added. "Everything else these days comes from China."

Ini yelped as he manipulated her leg.

"This dog come from the Rez?" he asked.

That's right, I responded, and added about how the hunter (whose dog attacked Ini) thought she was a coyote.

"Could be," he responded, his expression serious. "You never know what you gonna get out there. The dogs are kinda like the people – They're a different breed..."

CHAPTER SIXTEEN

As Ini underwent surgery, Somay and I sat in the waiting area.

"I'd seen you before with your dog," she said. "You'd be walking in front of the house, and there'd be this furry creature hopping behind you between snowdrifts... I would watch you guys out of the window, and the snow was higher than she was, so she would hop after you – She would pop out into the air to manage the snow being too high, so that she would hop, hop, hop, hop... That's when she was really small and the two of you would be going through the snow."

I asked where she lived?

"In the property just before the hills," she responded.

I nodded. Yes, Ini and I would go through there often.

I leaned back, remembering the moment I'd lifted Ini after the hunter's dog attacked her and the bond I felt with her.

"In my tradition there's a saying," I confided. "'He who saves a single life, saves the world.' My whole life I'd resisted that statement... Saving one life was never enough for me. I wanted to reach the millions."

I shook my head.

"But looking into Ini's eyes at that moment," I continued. "Seeing her in all that pain and agony – I had this feeling like the very reason I was put in this world was to help her."

"Are you Jewish, Dr. Mike?" she asked. "When I was at Amherst, I applied for a program about genocide that was sponsoring college students to go to the Auschwitz concentration camp. I was accepted for the program, and was the only non-Jewish member of the group. When we got to the camp, the moment that we crossed under that gate, I cried and cried. Even though I wasn't Jewish, I could feel the spirits of the dead crying out. Walking by the barracks, I was hearing the screams. Just all the suffering of those who perished there."

Most of my wife's family were murdered in Auschwitz. Indeed, April's grandparents missed being Holocaust victims themselves by the slimmest of margins – getting out of Czechoslovakia just before the Nazis invaded that nation and the border were closed. April had wanted to visit Auschwitz herself, but her grandmother forbade it – saying that all she'd find there was graves.

April's grandmother had died shortly after we married, and April was still grieving. By coincidence, Amherst College was located where April's grandparents first settled after they emigrated to this country – Northampton – and where April's mother was born.

"We learn that the Jewish people were expelled from their land and persecuted for thousands of years," Somay said. "But they stayed faithful to their ways and finally got their homeland back."

I turned my head.

"Have you been to Israel?" she asked.

Yes, I lived there for a year, I responded. My wife grew up in Israel.

"I heard your prayer for your wife," she commented.

I looked at her, surprised.

"During the ceremony," she added. "In the sweat lodge."

I hadn't realized she was there.

"Is she doing better?" she asked.

Yes, I said, curtly. Thanks for asking.

"How long have you been married, Dr. Mike?" she asked.

Not long - About a year, I responded.

It was actually considerably less than that.

"We'd known each other longer than that," I continued, absently. "We met thirteen years before. I was studying cancer vaccines at the National Institutes of Health, and she was doing an externship at the Smithsonian. There were reasons we didn't pursue each other. Years later, after a lot of failed relationships, I wrote her, and we got back together."

Somay nodded.

"So,   it   was   a   lesson   learned,"   she   said...

CHAPTER SEVENTEEN

The veterinarian reappeared and approached us.

"The dog tolerated the procedure," he said. "She's resting comfortably now. I'd suggest that you leave your dog here overnight, and I'd discourage you from visiting your pet right now. Dogs are usually quite attached to their owner. When an owner comes, the dog will cry and whine like it's being abandoned, and that won't do it any good..."

In the parking lot Somay gave me her number.

"If you need any help with Ini, you could give me a call," she said...

During the night I tossed in bed, playing over and over the day's events in my head.

She was doing so well, I thought. It was all going so well. I'll probably never see her hop that way again. How could I let this happen? Why did I take her there?

"Mike, from what you've told me, Ini loves going with you," April said. "She loves the car. She loves doing those long walks with you. She doesn't want to be separated from you. She's happy with you."

I didn't even know what was wrong with her. She just seemed plastered to where that other dog had pounced on her. It wasn't until the pitiful hobbling that I knew. She didn't come back to life again until we ran into Somay. She trusted Somay. I'd failed her.

"I'm pretty sure she came from the back of Somay's car to the front because she felt lonely, and needed some reassurance," April said. "She didn't need to do that with you because you were able to hold her. You were able to just be there and hold her. Somay wasn't able to concentrate on her because she needed to drive. Do you hear me, Mike?"

Yeah, I hear you, I said.

"But what you don't know is Ini moved away from me," I added. "When my arms got tired and I laid her down, she got up – in all that pain – and went under the brush. She wanted to get away from me. She wanted to find some place to crawl under and die."

"Mike, you're having bad thoughts," she said.

"It's the truth," I responded.

"No, it's not, it's not," she said, comfortingly. "It had nothing to do with you being selfish. It was about us being separated and this beautiful being coming into your life. I think Ini loves the time with you. The two of you were just out, hiking around, having fun. She got injured because another dog attacked her. That's all. It had nothing to do with you being selfish."

"Think about it, Mike," she continued. "When you brought Ini home, I asked you, 'If the dog jumped on you, would you have taken her home?' The answer was no. It took the dog to lie on top of your clothes and then lie in the snow before you took her home. Because you thought she needed you. Not because you wanted or needed a dog. It was because you didn't think she would be okay without you.

"Ini did the same thing when she broke her leg and crawled under the bush. She accepted her fate. And then you saved her again.

"You're always doubting yourself, Michael. You never feel like you do enough for people, but, really, you never quit trying to help them. Perhaps, a lovely being like Ini was brought into your life to try to teach you that.

"So stop blaming yourself. She just got hurt. It could have happened anywhere. It was just an unfortunate incident. A pure accident. You were not being selfish.

"Kids get hurt on the playground, for God's sake. I was just reading about how kids wind up with broken bones just coming down the slide. And it's mostly when the parents have been overprotective and gone down the slide with them that there leg gets caught, and the kid can't shift it. It almost never happens when they're on their own. But when they're on their parents overprotective laps – thinking they're doing the right thing for their children and protecting them – if their leg gets caught, they can't adjust the weight of the parent, and it keeps the momentum going, and they end up breaking their leg.

"The article said that the kids always recover fine, but what they did find was problems with the adult. The adult eats themselves up and gets very depressed, or the spouse gets very angry, and sometimes there's these severe marriage problems. That's usually the real problem with those injuries.

"And it all comes from the parents wanting to protect their kids – just be good to their kids – and they didn't know the danger. Like you – you didn't know..."

CHAPTER EIGHTEEN

In the morning there was a knock at the door; gazing through the peep-hole, Orville was standing on the porch.

"Dr. Mike, I'm sorry to hear about your puppy," he said. "Somay told me what happened. During the deer season, those hunters from town come to the Reservation with their guns and their dogs, and they hunt our game. We put signs up - 'No hunting' - but they come anyways. Sometimes, they pull down the signs. Then, they come to the casino at night and hit on our women. Anyway, it's unfortunate what happened to Ini. I hope she'll be up and around soon."

He kneeled and prayed over Ini. Afterward, he rose stiffly and turned to go. Then, he stopped and looked back.

"Our ways tell us that when a dog gets hurt, it was meant for the person," he continued. "She has a good heart. She sacrificed herself for you... Maybe, because you're hurting over something and don't even know it. Have a deep wound somewhere that she was sent to heal..."

CHAPTER NINETEEN

Arriving at the pet hospital the following morning, the office still hadn't opened. I walked to the town square, and took a seat in the breakfast shop. At the next table a man sat hunched and silent, looking old and stifled; stuck and stopped; as though not able to get out of a certain situation. Receding hairline, gray not unlike mine, he never smiled, not even a crack. Tired, unhappy, like there was nothing to look forward to; nothing to kindle that spark of life. Devoid of interest and excitement. Dead inside. Unable to get out of some unhappy place he found himself. No way out. Brows straight across and pointed downward, so that if you could have drawn a line across them, they would have intersected each other like an 'X' across his face.

Like he was locked in, I thought. Going through the motions. Eating, but seeming as though the food was devoid of flavor. He motioned to his wife that he was done, then left. Following his steps I wondered that I hadn't been treated to a glimpse of my future?

Walking through a residential neighborhood, a cat approached me on the sidewalk and rubbed against my left; I bent low and stroked its fur. Just then, a man appeared across a fence.

"What are you doing with that cat?" he said.

His question surprised me.

"You heard me," he demanded. "I said, 'What are you doing with that cat?'"

"I'm petting it," I responded.

"Well, I don't want you near that cat," he said. "I want you to stay away from that cat. Where did you say you're going?... The vet's. Well, that's a block away. Look, I can see you're just an animal lover, but I want you to stay away from that cat. If you start petting the can, that cat is going to try following you, till it crosses the street and gets hit by a car. So, stay away from that cat."

"Yeah, sure," I said. "I don't want any harm to come to your cat. Last thing I'd want."

I   turned   and   walked   away…

CHAPTER TWENTY

Returning to the pet hospital, a vet tech took me back to see Ini. Confined to a kennel, there was what looked like a lampshade strapped over her head.

"We had to place a Victorian collar on her to keep her from licking the wound," the tech said.

Though bleary eyed and tired, she flipped her tail the moment our eyes met.

"Ini is a trooper," the assistant said. "Okay, we need to give you a shot, darling."

Carrying a syringe towards Ini, the assistant turned to me.

"It's going to burn, so you better hold her," she said.

The tech gave the shot; Ini yelped, but a moment later, turned and licked the tech.

"I think you should call her, 'Special Forces,'" the tech said. "Because that dog doesn't let anything get her down for long."

Ini got up and limped towards me, dragging her injured leg. She appeared full of joy despite being near completely incapacitated. I knelt, looking into her soft brown eyes.

"Whoever questioned whether an animal had a soul must have never looked into the eyes of a dog," I said. "It makes me think of what the Lakota say in their ceremonies. *Mitakuye Oyasin*. 'We're all related.'"

"I don't believe that," the tech said. "The Bible tells us that man has dominion over the animals. All the creatures of the earth and sky. That's what the Good Book teaches us…"

CHAPTER TWENTY-ONE

The veterinarian entered the room and slapped a post-op X-ray on the light-box.

"The pin placement is good, but you'll have to confine the dog for a while," he said. "A kennel is best for three-to-four weeks. The dog can still break the pin if she goes to jumping, even in a small bathroom or utility room."

Inspecting the radiograph, it appeared the pin was protruding into the joint space.

"I had to leave it in the joint like that because the dog is still growing," he said. "A cast isn't needed, but she'll have to be kept in a splint. And just kennel rest. When she needs to go, put a leash on her and walk her out. She can stretch her legs for five-to-ten minutes, three-to-five times a day at slow pace. We'll plan on removing the pin in four-to-six weeks."

I nodded.

"So, you work for the Indians, huh?" he continued. "I prefer not to have much to do with anyone with an animal in any part of their name. Not very reliable, if you know what I mean."

Looking at me, he smiled.

"You might think about yourself, Doc," he said. "Do what's in your best interest. Take care of the ones who have the means to take care of you. The hospital here in town is looking for a Doc. I can introduce you to the Chief of Staff."

I'll give it some thought, I responded, blithely. He depressed the corners of his lips, and nodded towards the ground.

"You married, Doc?" he asked. "You might think twice about the way you're carrying on with that Indian girl. People around here talk. That includes folks on the Rez. What you do one minute, everyone will know about half an hour later."

He swung the door open to leave, then stopped and turned back.

"I don't totally agree with what the government did to the Indians," he said. "But if you look at history, in every age – and I don't care whether it was the Greeks or the Jews or the Babylonians or the Romans or Egyptians or whatever – when one culture conquered another, the conquered people had to adapt to the conqueror's ways. They had to find a way to get along and assimilate and survive in the conqueror's culture. That's just understood. That's what   conquered   people   do…"

CHAPTER TWENTY-TWO

Ini's in her kennel. For the past week she's compliantly laid there, day in and day out. The only time she's let out is so she can relieve herself. That's a sad spectacle – She hobbles around in the yard till she finds a place, and then it's right back in the kennel again...

Gazing up from my diary, I looked down at Ini. She responded by flipping her tail.

Stepping outside on the porch for some air, Ryan pulled up in his truck.

"How's it going, Doc?" he said. "How's Ini?"

"She's in the crate," I responded. "Kind of difficult to look at."

"Yeah," he said. "Hard to be without your companion, huh?"

His tone was slow and reassuring. I nodded. Then, from inside, I heard a pitiful groan, and excused myself to go back inside. Ryan lowered his head.

"Sure, Doc," he said.

Entering the room I knelt at the kennel, and inserted my fingers between the bars to stroke Ini's paw. Then, opening the cage, I crawled   inside,   and   laid   down   with   her...

CHAPTER TWENTY-THREE

On the day of Ini's follow-up appointment with the Vet, I was swamped with patients at the clinic, and called Somay to ask if she could take Ini?

"No problem, Dr. Mike," she said.

I met her at the house.

"Com' on, Ini," she said. "Let's see if they can take out that pin."

Lifting Ini into the car, she was wagging her tail as I closed the door...

In the afternoon Somay called from the pet hospital.

"They took out the pin," she said. "But the Vet said there's something about Ini's joints he has to talk with you about... That they're not working right..."

CHAPTER TWENTY-FOUR

"While your dog was still under, I tested the mobility in the joints," the Vet said. "None of the joints are moving properly. All that blood mixed with the muscles, tendons, and ligaments, and everything got scarred down. You could try exercises and stretching, but it probably won't change it. The joints are all locked up…"

As the days passed Ini continued to hobble on the injured leg.

"She doesn't want to do the stretching," I told April. "She pulls away from me every time I try."

"They probably hurt and she doesn't know why you're doing these things to her," April responded.

I nodded, remembering what it was like when I had to do undergo treatment for my leg – and I knew what it was for!

"I think it's okay, Mike," she said. "There's no real harm that comes from something done with love…"

CHAPTER TWENTY-FIVE

Returning to the veterinarian, I was hopeful he might offer some words of encouragement. But as he watched me walk with Ini to the examination room, he stood shaking his head.

"Yeah, the dog's getting around," he said, "but, mostly, she's hopping like a bunny. The joints are shot. If you keep letting her go around like that, she's just going to get worse..."

CHAPTER TWENTY-SIX

Arriving home I lifted Ini out of the car. Setting her down, she limped worse than before, entirely unwilling to put weight on the affected leg. As she hobbled around following me inside the house, I had the feeling like being haunted by a kindly spirit.

A knock came from the door.

"Hi Dr. Mike," Orville said. "My daughter said you went to see the vet again. How's Ini?"

I invited him inside.

"She isn't getting better," I responded. "The vet said her knee and ankle are shot, and she's only getting worse."

I hesitated.

"He said all I'm doing is prolonging the agony," I continued, "and I should let him amputate, or put her down. Anything else is selfish."

"Oh, well, let's take a look at her," he said. "See if it's all that bad."

Orville got down on the floor with Ini; gently lifting her limbs one at a time, he hummed and sang in Lakota.

"You have to allow the four-legged to challenge herself," he said, rising from the ground. "You have to take her to the natural places and let her instincts guide her - inspire her to push herself, and use the leg, use the muscles. Otherwise, the problems will set in and then she   will   be   in   pain..."

CHAPTER TWENTY-SEVEN

Orville left, and I did as he suggested.

But Ini continued to limp.

It's no use, I thought. She isn't getting better.

Later, there was another knock on the door. This time it was Somay.

"Dad said you came back from the vet's and that he gave you bad news," she said.

I nodded. But rehashing events at the veterinarian office, it struck me that not so long ago, doctors had made similar pronouncements about me.

"When I was at the National Institutes of Health," I said, "I hurt my leg. I went to all kinds of doctors – Sports Medicine specialists, Orthopedists, Neurologists. They told me I just had to accept that I wouldn't walk normally again, and I'd be in constant pain."

"But you walk okay, Dr. Mike," Somay said. "What did you do?"

I made a thorough study of my condition, and learned about a technique called ischemic compression used for treating muscle spasms.

All muscles have a central artery moving through them. Spasms constrict the artery, so that blood supply is compromised. By applying pressure to those muscles, you restrict the blood flow even further, so that the spasm will either release, or the pain will be such that you won't be able to tolerate the treatment. It was a long process, but for the most part, it worked.

"Could you do that on Ini?" she asked.

I shook my head. The vet said the problem's in the joints, I responded. Not the muscles.

"Was he sure?" she asked. "It doesn't mean you can't try."

Nodding, I remembered my friend, Ethel. Diagnosed with pancreatic cancer, she suffered intense back pain. I was a medical student at the time, and sure the pain was because of the cancer. Unlike other cancers that just expand against the nerves, this one infiltrated the nerve sheathes, attacking the raw nerve endings, and caused the worst pain known to medicine – worse than kidney stones. The only treatment was high dose narcotic pain medicine, and hope the cancer would quickly ran its course.

But the pain was becoming unbearable; even with the high dose narcotics, she was still suffering.

Finally, I examined her; muscles in her back were in spasm, so I decided to try ischemic compression. When I did, the spasms melted away under my fingertips – even with the slightest of pressure. It was great - and horrible... Great because it gave her so much relief; horrible because I'd waited so long.

"Try it on Ini," Somay said. "Why don't you try?"

I examined Ini. The muscles were taut - in such spasm so to deform the leg. I applied gentle pressure. But Ini whimpered and raised her head. She put her head down, and I tried again. This time, she seemed to indicate pain by raising her tail, and then thumping it down.

She doesn't know what I'm doing, I thought. Sometimes, the knots don't come out right away and the technique can be painful. I don't think I can do it on her.

"I'll hold her," Somay said.

Somay stroked Ini's head.

"Ini, do you remember when you hurt your leg?" she said. "The bone is all better, but your muscles are still hurt, and daddy's trying to make the muscles better by hurting them temporarily. Do you think you can understand that?"

I thought it was silly. But Ini relaxed under Somay's touch, and I applied pressure. A knot in her leg jumped suddenly, then dissolved under my fingertips. Several more followed. It felt like a proverbial 'bag of worms', the muscle bands writhing and twisting, till melting away. The leg lost its contorted, twisted shape; when Ini got up, she walked without limping.

"I think she's walking a lot better," Somay said. "She's not favoring the bad leg as much."

Ini was putting her weight on the injured leg again.

"You see, you did it," Somay said. "You don't have to go back to that vet again. You and Ini don't need him anymore..."

CHAPTER TWENTY-EIGHT

With time Ini recovered her athleticism. The leg still displayed some turnout – like a ballet dancer doing a plie – though when we'd walk along the train tracks and she would move her legs in perfect tandem.

Healing is a life-long commitment, I thought. Things in life happen. But where there exists the possibility of healing, it might be worth it to not give up. Because you never know what may lay ahead – healing, love, joy, friendship. It takes effort. But if you're willing to try, there might yet be some light.

My tranquil thoughts were interrupted by a rustling in the brush. A large deer leapt out, and Ini ran after it in head-long pursuit. I called her, but to no avail. When I caught up with her, she was limping.

She'd pushed her abilities too far, too fast, I thought.

The walk home was painful, as she limped, and at times trotted on three legs.

Then, during the night Ini was like a little jumping bean, repeated racked by spasms that shook her whole body, in and out of sleep. I lay holding her as the spasms seemed to rip through her dreams. But in the morning Ini woke up spry, running around and appearing better than ever...

"It reminded me of the movie *What about Bob?*" I told Somay. "In the movie a psychiatrist gets so fed up with a patient, he straps him to a bomb, and tells him if he can't undo all the knots at once, he'll explode."

Somay laughed.

"That's what it was like last night," I said. "Ini was undoing all these knots at once. It was like watching her undue herself with each round of dreams."

Ini was teaching me new exercises, as well; as she bit at my heel, I'd pivot in place, and chase her, round-and-round.

"By circling me this way," I said, "she exercises the abductor and adductor muscles of her leg. While stuck in that kennel recuperating, the muscles of the leg had wasted to next to nothing. This kind of exercising was rebuilding them."

Somay examined the muscles in Ini's leg.

"You're right," she said. "I can feel the muscles are bigger now."

"But it's more than just Ini," she added. "You're walking better, too. You're not walking with as much of a limp."

I looked at her, quizzically.

"Ini limps on the same leg that you have problems with," Somay said.

I depressed the corners of my lips.

I guess were birds of a feather, I said. Or dogs of a feather – though including me this way might be offensive to the *Shunka* [Dog] Nation.

"Maybe you can heal like her," Somay tells me you have a wound," he said. "She said she worked on it. She said. "You can heal together…"

CHAPTER TWENTY-NINE

During the night Ini growled in her sleep; harsh, wolf-like snarls that accompanied a series violent jumping of the muscles in her legs, as though releasing some savage wolfian being.

Examining Ini I found some residual spasms, though most were in the unaffected leg?!

Probably from compensating, I thought.

The overall muscle mass of the left leg still felt smaller, probably enfeebled by the months of lack of use. I felt at my own leg, and considered the accident that had happened to me as a child.

An occasional whimper rose up in between the muscular twitches in her legs and back. Imagining she was in the throes of a nightmare, I quietly laid down next to her, and stroked her fur.

"Don't worry," I whispered. "Daddy's here."

The words kindled thoughts about my father. How could he leave us? A wife and two little boys? How had it been that he was able to not be there for us?

I considered his own childhood, raised by a father with untreated manic-depression.

I can't fault him, I thought. It must have been like living with a mad man. He'd had to do everything for himself. How would he know how to be supportive?

The twitches become fewer, and Ini's muscles relaxed.

If you give someone – or some thing – some support, I reflected, they're going to get through it. They're going to heal and get to a better place.

And maybe sometimes we have to find good parents outside of our biological ones? Sometimes we need to go to someone else – a therapist – trained in how to give support. So we need others at times to step up and provide support. Those who know how to be supportive. To give what others can't because they're victim to significant historical trauma.

I thought about my patients. As children a lot of them were taken away from their families, away from their tribes, away from everything they knew, and brutalized. What do they know about giving love and support?

"You may not realize it," a patient told me, "but you're really peaceful, and I like that. You don't argue, nothing, you just speak. Sometimes, I'll get back from seeing you, and I'll read the instructions you've written out for me about how to exercise the muscles in my hand, and I'll turn it back to page one and just keep reading again till I go to sleep.

"Because when I back up, I don't even have a problem starting over. It's kind of one of them deals that I enjoy the instructions. So thank you. Thank you for sending me home with them."

People and things need restful sleep to heal. Sleeping and dreaming are a time when we work through a lot of our problems. I thought about my patients plagued with nightmares, so that they were deprived of that restful, healing sleep.

Part of rest is feeling trust, I thought. Feeling like you can cope with a nightmare.

"Yeah," he'd said. "Some people have comfort pillows and whatever. I used to sleep with a 45 under my pillow, just because I was afraid someone was going to murder me in my sleep. But no more 45. I have Dr. Mike's instructions..."

Nodding off, I dreamt I saw Stan in a river, effortlessly moving against the current. All that strength, I thought. In no time – in the span of a few long, steady strides – he was gone.

Awakening, I found Ini, still asleep, had turned towards me, so that she was draped over my left shoulder; her paws flaring in and out across my chest, as though she were reaching to my heart. Then, the left shoulder – the one I typically have problems with at the end of the day – underwent a massive twitch, the muscles releasing.

That's funny? I thought...

At Somay's, we positioned Ini to perform ischemic compression. Ini looked up at Somay and beat her tail against the floor.

"You're so pretty when you smile," Somay said. "You're always pretty, but you make my heart sing when you smile."

There seemed so many injured muscles; surprisingly, the knots released easily under slight pressure.

"I wish knots came out of me so easily," I said. "In the past, doctors had to needle me to get the spasms out."

"How about stretching?" she asked.

I shook my head.

"I've tried that, but it really doesn't do much for me," I said. "Ischemic compression is what's worked."

"I can work on your leg, Dr. Mike," she said. "I see you limp. It looks like it's hurting you."

I positioned myself next to Ini, and Somay applied pressure along the injured muscles.

"Wow," Somay said. "The bands in your legs are just like Ini's. It's funny... It's the same leg as Ini's. Like it's the same muscles."

When I was perhaps eight or nine years old, I was hit by a car. It crippled the left leg. Twenty years later I injured the right one, and with neither leg to rely on, I couldn't ignore the injury anymore.

As Somay applied pressure, I winced and pulled away.

"Now you know how Ini feels," she said. "And she can't even say, 'That hurts. It's bothering me. Can you be more gentle there?'"

As she worked on the muscles, my thoughts drifted to my patient with knee pain; how difficult it was for him to walk; how painful it was; did he have someone to help him the way Somay was helping me? I couldn't even get him physical therapy!

Ini moved in and nudged Somay's hand; she laughed.

"Don't worry, Ini," she said. "Daddy's getting ischemic compression, too..."

CHAPTER THIRTY

"Dr. Mike, I have a liniment that I think will be good for you," Somay said. "I made it from white clover I found in Spring Creek. Can I use it on your leg?"

She went to her dresser.

"When I was growing up, I'd gather plants and stuff with my grandma. All the good things they do for us. Sometimes I want to write a book. I don't want to lose these plants. Nobody's interested in them. 'It's too hard.' 'I don't want to have to dig.' 'I don't want to sweat.' 'Can't I just buy something at the store?' My own people have come up with a hundred excuses why not to save plants. I'm not even that old, and I'm a fossil, Dr. Mike. But I'm not going to give up. That's why I need to put it in book form, so that later on it doesn't end up that all these things just wind up in a museum. 'Oh yeah, they used to collect plants...' You know, I don't want that to happen. There's got to be somebody.

"Sometimes I identify these things in a book. And I think to myself, 'Oh my God. My grandmother knew this. How did she know about this stuff?' It's such a shock that my grandmother would know such wondrous things.

"I don't know. She never sat down for a meal with a white person in her life. But she knew so much. I'm blown away by it. And all the things they talk about with my grandmother, and why she did it, and how fun it was to gather plants with her. I never did complain about sitting in the sun, or sweating. Because, boy, grandma made it fun. She even showed me how to make Indian shampoo and soap. All kinds of good things."

As Somay worked the liniment into the knotted muscles of my leg, my thoughts drifted to my mother.

"Funny the things that run through your mind at times," I said. "My mother told me, 'I only had a teddy bear growing up; I never had a doll. Can you believe that?' 'What's so hard to believe?' I said. 'Because I always wanted a doll,' she said, 'and never had one.' I asked if she wanted me to go out and get her one? Like the time she took me to the store to get that mechanical toy dog."

I hesitated.

"My mother hurt her leg doing ballet," I continued. "She was never the same after that... She never got better. She spent the rest of my childhood in bed writhing in pain."

When I was hit by that car, my mom took me to the Emergency Room. There weren't any broken bones, but, after, I couldn't do the things I used to. Couldn't skate. Couldn't run fast, or in a straight line.

"Did the car drive over you?" Somay asked.

No, it just knocked me into the street. As I lay on the ground, the driver repeated, "Bad boy. Bad boy."

"Why did he say that?"

I couldn't be sure; maybe it was because I'd been riding on the sidewalk.

"In the end," I said, "it was my fault."

Somay was quiet.

"I won't let my nephew Wesley ride his bike on the street," she said. "The streets aren't safe. The police could ticket Wesley for riding on the sidewalk as much as they want. But I don't ever want to receive a call or see the appearance of the police at my door because Wesley was run down. I just couldn't deal with that."

I looked on, doubtful.

The law is the law, I thought...

CHAPTER THIRTY-ONE

Arriving home Ini lay with her head resting near me and fell into a deep sleep, breathing softly against my shoulder.

Our ways tell us that when a dog gets hurt, it was meant for the person.

Maybe, this dog was meant to break a cycle of injury? I thought.

I recalled how our lives intersected; she at the Sweat Lodge, falling back in the snow; seemingly ready to surrender any hope of life. That had happened to me: When I was perhaps seven or eight years old, I'd been riding the waves at the beach in New York, when I got caught in an undertow, and I couldn't get out. Tossed over and over in the water, I finally stopped struggling. And in that moment – when I'd surrendered my fate – I experienced a calm, and feeling of inner peace and tranquility like none I'd ever known...

In the morning Orville appeared at my home.

"My daughter tells me you have a wound," he said. "She said she worked on it. She has a gift. Some people call it a 'power.' But it's not really a power; it's a gift that a man or a woman receives, and they use these gifts to work with people's needs and to help people many different ways – physically or lifestyle. These people are known as medicine men – and women. They have several names in that role. *Pejuta wicasa. Pejuta* is medicine, but it fits more for an herbalist - people who work with herbs, plants - people who are gifted to do that. My daughter has that gift. She makes cough syrups, lotions, and things like that..."

CHAPTER THIRTY-TWO

Your religion was written on tables of stone by the iron finger of an angry God, so you would not forget it. The red man could never understand it or remember it. Our religion is in the ways of our forefathers, the dreams of our old men, sent them by the Great Spirit, and the visions of our sachems. And it is written in the hearts of our people.
~ Chief Seattle

April was flying in. Driving through the Badlands on the way to the airport, I pulled over, and Ini and I got out and walked amongst the striated canyons and gullies. To the west there was an approaching storm, so that the skies in that direction were almost pitch black; but to the East the sun shone brightly, illuminating the Badland spires like beacons of light.

If you want great spirituality, you have to get connected to the Great Spirit.

As I stood pondering the message of the voice in my head, I recalled the conversation with Orville, about the nature of Lakota spirituality, and my disbelief that a culture built on an oral tradition could arrive at such an advanced way of thinking. Now, I understood. The answer was simple. The key was being connected.

Mitakuye   Oyasin,   I   said.   We   are   all   related...

CHAPTER THIRTY-THREE

At the airport April was waiting at the curbside. Pulling alongside her, she peered through the passenger window at Ini.

"What a beautiful girl?!" she said to Ini's delight. "Who is this beautiful girl?!"

Opening the door, Ini scampered towards April, characteristically wagging her entire body.

"She's so wiggly," she said. "It's not even just her tail – her whole body wiggles. She's like, 'Hello, play with me. There's nothing better in the whole world right now than me hanging out with you.'"

Driving to the Reservation, April stroked Ini's fur.

"She's so soft," she said.

April laid her long hair lengthwise against Ini.

"Ini and I have the same color hair," she said. "I guess you like girls with our coloring."

"Look, Ini's smiling," she continued. "She's got the cutest smile. I swear – I've never seen a dog smile so bright.

"Just before I came here, I was telling my niece the story about how we had to stop trying to get pregnant and you adopted Ini, and before I could finish it, she goes, 'Does that mean that Ini and Socks are my cousins?' Isn't that sweet? She got it. She totally got it. These are our kids..."

Arriving at the house Ini stayed close to April's side.

"It looks like Ini is keeping an eye on me," April said. "I guess I'm the lost sheep."

"She really is special," she continued. "The way she moves. The way she nuzzles."

Yes, I said. A pure gift.

"Don't forget," she added. "She was a gift to me."

Yes. Gift from the spirits...

CHAPTER THIRTY-FOUR

Driving through the Reservation, April expressed surprise.

"I was expecting wide-open spaces without a lot of trees because of the wind here," she said. "But there are a lot of trees because of the valleys here."

Arriving at the house I suggested a walk. Venturing into the seemingly endless expanse of open plains beyond the medical complex, Ini trotted off and seemed to disappear and vanish into high grass.

"She blends perfectly into the surroundings," April said. "She's a dog that looks like grass."

Returning, Ini stopped next to April with what appeared a big smile on her face.

"She's such a happy doggie," April said. "She tells you she's happy with her whole body. She has a spring in her step, and she stands stately and tall. And she's so graceful. She puts out her paws just so."

Content, Ini trotted off again, her right ear flopping, while the other remained upright.

"Those ears of hers are really cute," April said. "With the one she has up and the other down, it's like she's telling you, 'I'm a rascal.'"

Ini sniffed at something in the grass, then got on her back and shifted back and forth.

"Probably, some deer poop," April said. "Rubbing it into her fur, so she can disguise her scent and sneak up things." Then, in a deep, menacing tone added, "The better to eat you, my boy."

That's really what you think? I said.

"Of course," she responded. "So she can sneak up on unsuspecting prey."

April eyed Ini with interest.

"She has the coat of a German Shepherd," she said. "But her body type looks more like a greyhound.

"And her size is more a border collie's. And she's smart like a border collie."

"I always knew Ini was smart, though," she continued. "Because she knew the one thing she could do that would get you to bring her home... Lying on your clothes that night you found her. You wouldn't have brought her home if she'd just jumped on you, or licked your leg. But asleep on your clothes at night in the snow, and there was no way you were going to leave her - you were going to take that puppy home."

"She did a guilt trip on you," she concluded. "'I'm going to die if you don't take me.'"

April knelt and pet Ini.

"My little Cinderella who began her life a homeless Rez dog," she said. "I think even then she already knew she wanted to be a Jewish princess..."

At the house April went to the computer.

"When you originally sent me that picture of Ini," she began, "I looked up on the Internet about the dogs that Native Americans used to have – before they were displaced by the European dogs that were brought into this country. Ini looks a lot like those Indian dogs. She might have a lot of Indian dog in her. She doesn't really look like anything else. She might be part German Shepherd – part border collie. But, really, she doesn't resemble any particular breed. She might really be a good part Indian dog."

April brought up images of native dogs. In one photo taken with a Lakota warrior taken in the 1800s, there was a dog that looked exactly like Ini.

"That's probably why it's been hard to place her," April said. "The Indian dog breed is very rare today."

"It makes sense," she continued. "Why wouldn't she be an Indian dog? Or at least have some of that in her? I'm sure she's got the other stuff in her, too. I'm sure she's part border collie and German shepherd and all of that. But I think she's got some Native American in her, too.

"Many dogs came from England and bred with the Indian dogs that were here. Some were bred to defend their owners against wild boars and bears - And not back down. I think Ini would do that. Just the look in her eyes and the love she has for you, I don't think she would let anybody ever hurt you."

"I think you have a dog for life," she concluded. "This dog will live with you and stay beside you till the day she die – Because that's just her breed..."

CHAPTER THIRTY-FIVE

In the morning I didn't see Ini in the yard. Going outside, though, April and I found her playing with Bright Eyes on the other side of the fence.

"There's a hole at the corner," April said. "I guess Ini dug her way through to her friend."

Ini and Bright Eyes raced up and down the yard; low to the ground, digging into the ground, Ini ran like the wind; Bright Eyes couldn't keep up.

"Where other dogs seem to be running at full throttle, Ini just puts it in another gear and leaves them in the dust," April said. "It's like a standard car trying to compete with a Ferrari."

April eyed Ini closer.

"I think Ini's part greyhound," she said. "If you look at the arch of her back, and the tight way she holds her abdomen, that's like a greyhound."

Looking on I marveled at how far Ini had come – from a broken creature (one that had seemingly given up on life at the time of the injury) to the one running and interacting with her fellow creatures with a joy that could only come from being in the land of the living.

"It doesn't look like she has a limp," April said. "If you didn't know what happened to her, no one would ever know."

Ryan appeared on his porch rubbing his hands together.

"Brrr, kind of cold," he said. "Geez, if it's gonna be thirty-two degrees, there could at least be snow, huh? That's the old man from the north keeping everyone humble."

I introduced April, and she apologized to Ryan for the hole Ini dug into his backyard.

64

"Of course, Mike pay's no mind to that kind of thing," she said. "Ini has Mike wrapped around her little paw. He does not like when anyone says anything's wrong with his little puppy. He just let's her do anything she wants."

"Dr. Mike sure was worried about her the times he couldn't find her," Ryan said. "It's just lucky Ini got to Dr. Mike before the cops found her. They shot all the dogs on the Reservation... They were all the stray dogs. After that case of rabies, there was just a pile of them behind the jail. Me and Bright Eyes saw them when we were taking a walk behind the ravine there. Every time I look at Ini, I think, 'She had maybe three days.' If she hadn't found Dr. Mike when she did, she would have been in one of those piles."

April turned to me.

"I wonder if Ini knows how lucky she is to have met you?" she asked. "If you hadn't taken her, she wouldn't have lived past two months."

I shrugged, saying I felt it was me who was the lucky one.

"We're lucky to have her, and she is lucky to have us," April responded. "Without you, she would have been at the bottom of that ravine."

Ryan watched the dogs play, admiringly.

"It looks like Ini's doing better," he said.

He eyed her closer. "I think she's like a combination of fox and German Shepherd."

"'Foxy shepherd'," April responded. "I like that. The prettiest shepherd that's ever been born."

Ryan turned to April.

"So, how are you liking it here?" he asked.

"I do," she responded. "I always wanted to be out here – ever since I worked at NMAI [National Museum of the American Indian]."

She laughed.

"Sorry, I was thinking of something my sisters told me just before the trip," she added. "They said, 'After all the Native American boyfriends you had, it took marrying a Jewish doctor to get you to the Reservation.'"

"Do you think you and the cat are coming out here any time soon?" Ryan asked.

"I can't for the time being," she responded. "I'm still getting treatment."

"I'm sorry to hear that," he said.

He looked down, then into the distance.

"So, you worked at NMAI," he said. "There are remains of an earth lodge a couple hours from here near the Missouri River. I've been wanting to give Dr. Mike a tour. Do you have some time for me to take you?..."

CHAPTER THIRTY-SIX

The earth lodges were round and domed.

"They were probably built by the Mandan or Arikara," Ryan commented.

"It's interesting that somebody lived in here at one point," April said.

"Yeah, they're pretty sturdy," he responded. "They couldn't survive the dam, though. The only reason this one's here is because it was built so high up. The others were carried away when the dam went up."

"I can still remember it," he continued. "I was a kid back then. I was helping out, working with the construction crew because it was the only work to be had back then. When a burial site was flooded – and all these body parts found floating around – that's when I gave them my notice and stopped working on it."

Then, he pointed to a cliff that rose hundreds of feet above the river.

"It's the only place where you can see the river on two sides," he said. "Lewis and Clark noted it in the expedition when they first encountered us. We can go up there if you like…"

The three of us made our ascent of the cliff above the hairpin turn in the river. Walking in single file, I was in the lead, with April just behind me and Ryan taking up the rear. Then, stepping atop the plateau, I heard a rustling in the brush, and two prairie grouse sprang out at once right in front of me – one of them flying straight at me.

Startled, I stepped back and stumbled on a rock, and instinctively reaching out for April as I nearly fell.

Ryan burst out laughing.

"I'm sorry, Doc," he said, trying to restrain himself. "It's just you looked so scared by those birds, it was like you went hiding behind your wife."

Still holding me, April laughed, too.

"I guess we'll remember this as the famous bird expedition," she said…

CHAPTER THIRTY-SEVEN

For lunch Ryan recommended a restaurant in the border town located in a marina just off the Missouri.

"They got hamburger for dogs," he said. "Ini will love it."

'Hamburger for dogs'? I repeated, unbelieving.

"Um-hum," he responded. "They actually advertise it. It's for two dollars. They don't put anything in it. I get it for my dogs all the time..."

Ini looked surprised at first when the server set the hamburger down for her, but after the initial shock, she consumed it with gusto.

"She did love it," April commented.

"I actually found that most places would do it," Ryan responded. "You just tell them, 'Do you hat have anything without any of the spices?' Just be sure to tell them, 'I don't want it raw.'"

Ini looked at us, smiling.

"I think the next time we come here, Ini's going to be like, 'Where is my hamburger?... Hey, I think I get a hamburger here, right?'..."

Before leaving, I announced I'd brought my inflatable kayak, and said I wanted to take it on the Missouri.

"I wouldn't recommend it, Dr. Mike," Ryan responded. "The Missouri can be pretty treacherous."

Still, I wanted to try, and after inflating it, set out for the river inlet.

But just as I did, a strong wind blew off the river, and as hard as a paddled, I kept being pushed back.

After several tries, I finally gave up, and returned to others, shamefaced.

"Well, your dog sure is happy that you're back," Ryan commented. "Did you hear her?... She was howling the whole time you were out there..."

In the evening, April and I took Ini for a walk. There was a gentle breeze that rustled the leaves of all the trees and bushes, and I commented to April how pleasant it was.

"Earlier in the day, you were annoyed by that wind," she responded. "You were trying to go into the Missouri River from the marina and the winds kept you from entering. It was like the Lakota saying, 'We want to keep you as our doctor. We don't want to see you swept into the river.'"

I nodded. Considering how much difficulty I had in the marina, I might have been in a 'whole heap of trouble' if I'd actually succeeded in entering the mighty Missouri.

Then, it struck me that that was something my beloved Lakota friend and artist, Lenny, would say, as I recalled the kind of euphemisms ("Mighty peaceful", etc.) he used to use.

I recalled meeting him at the Lakota Youth Center just after the suicide cluster on the Reservation and his efforts to help high-risk youth.

"He was like that wind," April said of him. "Trying to keep people from going out into the Missouri. But they keep going in there."

I asked what she meant?

"Well, that wind kept you in the lagoon or whatever," she explained. "It didn't let you go into the danger zone, where it was too deep and too powerful for you. For the Lakota people, it just feels like so many of them go into the river emotionally and get swept away and their life is shit."

I still wasn't sure – How were they going into the river?

"I don't know," she responded. "Alcohol. Drug use. Unemployment. All those things that they get swept up in. Lenny was trying to make tools for them, so that they didn't go in the river – and get swept away in the river. That was his big thing. To keep them from going in that river."

River of despair, I realized.

"Yep," she said. "Get them to learn how to make art. Make drums."

"But to keep them from going into the river is kind of like trying to hold off a flood," she lamented.

Were they like me? I asked. Approaching the Missouri like they thought it would be adventurous? Like it would be fun?

"No," she responded, softly. "It's like the healers that you interacted with told you... It's the effects of historical trauma – That caused their parents and grandparents to not have parents. And not know how to parent – So that they're all broken up."

"But you know that," she asserted, exasperated. "You've seen them in their worst moments... In the hospital and all that. You know what the Lakota are experiencing..."

CHAPTER THIRTY-EIGHT

Returning at the end of the work day, I opened the door to find Ini waiting with a stuffed animal.

"Did you see what she did?" April said, laughing. "When she saw you coming, she ran from outside to the door, and then she ran back to the kitchen and grabbed her fox, and then she stood there with the fox in her mouth, and started inviting you to go outside with her to play. She's so smart."

"Ini really misses you," she added. "She's like a different dog when you aren't around. That spark goes out after you leave the house and she kind of waits for you all day."

The stuffed animal still in Ini's mouth, she challenged me to take it from her.

Tommy Post, I thought aloud. God don't let me poke you, my sweet Tommy Post.

"Who's Tommy Post?" April asked.

Tommy Post was a boyhood friend. He was a fabulous athlete, and every time I'd lunge to get a stuffed animal away from Ini, I thought of him.

"Why?" she asked.

Because once while I was over Tommy's, he bet me a dollar I couldn't hit him with a ball as he leapt from the pool. Surfacing like a seal before diving back under water, he evaded my every throw.

Then, in frustration, I decided to aim for his head, and made contact with my first throw. It was terrible; his nose bled and bled.

And worst of all, true to his word, he went to his piggy bank and – still sobbing – gave me the dollar reward.

I shook my head.

"Can you imagine?" I asked. "Accepting money for intentionally hurting someone?"

Just then, as I was wrestling with Ini over the stuffed animal, she lifted her head and smacked me full on the mouth.

"Uh-oh," April uttered.

I just smiled.

That's good, I thought, my lip swelling with the taste of blood. Thank you. God in your mercy, thank you – for clearing me of some of the bad karma from what I inflicted on Tommy.

Pulling Ini close, I looked up to the clear blue skies in the backdrop of April's laughter.

Thank you, Ini, I thought. Thank you, God...

The sweet smell of spring in the air, we walked out into the open Plains.

Ini seemed to sense something over a hill and went running until she was out of view. Then, I heard the sound of something screeching and went running after her.

A prairie dog mound came into view, and Ini trotting back with one of its members.

"Drop it!" I demanded.

Ini immediately complied – though her expression hinted at confusion.

With the exception of a few sporadic twitches, the prairie dog lay still.

"Probably, broke its neck," April commented. "That's usually how dogs kill smaller prey."

Nodding, I recalled the way Ini would shake her stuffed animals, and the image of Blackie the night he went after Foxie entered my head.

Why would she do it? I thought. She hadn't been chained or teased in any way?

"That's meat on a stick, Michael," April responded. "She's willing to share it with you. A hundred years ago that might have been a nice offering to cook over the fire."

I shook my head; I wasn't interested in any 'sharing'; I wanted her to leave the little creatures alone.

"You got yourself a little huntress," April responded. "She's got killer instincts. If that isn't what you want, you're going to have either train that out of her or not let her run wild..."

Poems by April.

Sometimes Ini is the thunder dog,
As she guards the backyard,
And thunders, "Mine, mine,"
Across the fence at the neighbor's dogs.
Sometimes Ini is the yelping dog.
Sometimes she's the silent one.
And sometimes she's nudging,
Nudging us with her soft muzzle.
Nudging, yelping, thundering doggie.
Who has brown eyes,
Soft and warm.

Waiting for rain
the lawn yellow
with bites of
green
hoping the rain will come
relieve the dry, choking thirst
the roses not blooming
the berries dry on the branches
the air nice and dry on my skin
not humid like
back east
where the forest lines the highway
with green
and the air is thick and sticky.

CHAPTER THIRTY-NINE

April told me that she and Ini had taken a walk earlier in the day and encountered a coyote along the way.

"When we saw that coyot', Ini made these sounds," she said. "She didn't bark. It wasn't the kind of sound she makes towards dogs. It was a growling. Maybe she could feel that coyot' didn't have good intentions. Maybe that's what it was?"

"Ini really does look like a coyot'," she continued. "The same color. The same size. When you look at her from far away, she really does look more like a coyot' than a dog. I can understand why the hunter mistook her for a coyot'. If you're not looking at the spirit and intention of the animal, they really do look similar."

Looking at Ini – smiling as she walked amidst the fields – all I could see was her beautiful spirit.

"And with the neighbor's cat, Ini is so amazing," April added. "Today, the cat came into the backyard and walked over Ini. The cat actually put its paws on Ini's side, jumps over her, then walks in between Ini's legs. And Ini doesn't flinch. She just laid there. She didn't move a muscle. It's crazy. She didn't growl. She made no sound. She just accepted it."

"I think she'll be good with Socks," she continued. "They both are very smart. You think that comes from being on their own in the beginning?"

I thought about how we'd acquired Socks – an abandoned kitten we'd taken in before a storm – and how similar it was to Ini.

"But I think with Socks it's very different," she said. "Socks is partly feral, but she's a lot more independent... I mean, thinking for herself - Needing freedom. I don't think of Ini that way..."

CHAPTER FORTY

April couldn't sleep and stayed up reading. Seeing as I had to be up early for morning rounds, I retired to the bedroom.

Ini followed me and lied curled at the foot of the bed. When April finally joined us, I went to hug her and (from behind) I felt Ini leave her curled position and straighten, so to lay vertical like the two of us.

Then, Ini placed a paw on my shoulder.

April laughed.

"It's like she is giving us her blessing," she said.

I turned to look, but April pulled me back.

"No, no," she said. "It's so seldom that we hold each other like this."

Ini kept her paw on my shoulder.

"Does it feel like she's pushing you?" April asked.

No, not pushing, I said. Just present there.

Finally, I turned. Ini licked me, then put her arm around me in a curled fashion like she was giving me a hug.

"She wants you to know that she loves you, too," she said. "She's staring into your eyes with love. Do you see that?... Oh, I love that girl. I just love that girl."

She reached over to pet Ini.

"What did we do to deserve a being like this?" she said. "Those must have been some really good prayers that the spirits blessed us this way. They heard them and decided those prayers were worthy. She decided your prayers were worthy..."

In the morning Ini lay above April in bed, her body curled around April's head like some living halo.

76

"How do you like my dog pillow?" April asked.

She stroked Ini's fur.

"How did we wind up winning the dog lottery?" she said.

She looked at me.

"Can you imagine if you didn't pick her up and take her up on her invitation?" she asked. "To perish by shooting?"

She petted Ini's forehead.

"Ini has such distinctive features," she said. "Eyebrows that aren't eyebrows. She has a heart right there on her forehead. You can't disguise who you are, Ini. You're a furry heart on four legs."

She snuggled Ini and referred to her as "honey."

"I mean, look at her," she exclaimed. "Isn't she a honey? Her coloring, her soft eyes. Everything about her is honey. All the different kinds of honey: She's dark honey, to light honey. She's all different amber colors. Honey!"

Then, April straightened, smiling.

"I've decided that dog-honey is a very good human-catcher," she continued. "I know what Ini is... She's a coyo-deer."

She laughed.

"Do you think those two could make a baby together?" she asked.

I shook my head, then kissed Ini.

"Goodbye my little coyo-deer," I said.

Then, April.

"And goodbye my other dear."

On the table I left a couple anniversary cards – one of them signed for Ini as well as me.

Returning home April and Ini were on the couch, smiling.

"When I opened the card, Ini was pretty close to me on the bed," April said. "So, I look up and she was looking right at me. So, I show her the card and said, 'That's from you to me.' And then, Ini licked it."

"Yeah, that was very sweet," she continued. "It was like I looked up and she was right there sitting next to me. I guess she knew. I guess she had a feeling about it. So, I really felt like she was giving me the card..."

Porcelain pink dress princess
broken into fragments
Best friend's stepdad
glued her back together
The break lines darkening over the years
the triangle hole with piece missing
Who thought
later on
She'd fix many ceramic objects
for a living...

CHAPTER FORTY-ONE

"What's this poem about?" I asked April. *"Porcelain pink dress princess'?...* What's the story behind it?"

"It was my favorite gift from my grandma," she responded. "A porcelain pink dress princess. She gave it to me as a present while I was visiting her when I was just six or seven. I took it back with me to Israel, and when it fell and broke, I was really broken up about it.

"So, my friend, Sharon, asked her stepdad to fix it, because he was always fixing things. And he fixed it. I was really touched by that.

"I actually have it. The glue is quite black now, and as a conservator, I really should redo it."

Why would you do that? I asked. It seemed to me that the most meaningful thing about the object now is the glue and the care that Sharon's stepfather put into fixing it.

"Yes!" she responded, spiritedly. "Yes. That's what they would teach us in Art Conservator School. 'Preserve the history of the object' – That there's beauty in the breaks!..."

We went outside with Ini.

"Ini says, 'I like it when dad comes home. He goes on a walk with us,'" April said. "You can see her say that in the way she holds herself – Tail up, body humming with excitement."

We crossed a path with high grass.

"Do you ever worry about snakes?" she asked. "I'm like terrified of them."

Perhaps an omission in my innate programming, I responded. Because I certainly wasn't particularly inclined to think about them; I was just enjoying the outdoors, the nature, the open fields, and there wasn't the lurking thought of what else could happen.

"Of the two of us, you're definitely more of the risk taker," she commented. "That's one of the personality traits that got them to pick me out to become an art conservator."

"I know to get into medical school it was really hard," she continued, "but it's also really hard to get into art conservation programs. The year that I applied, there were only three programs in the entire United States, and each one of them took just ten students. So there were thirty spots a year, and hundreds of people applying. So it wasn't so easy to get into, and they did lots of testing. It was a full day interview, and thinking ahead was one of the things they wanted. That and assessing risk – What could go wrong, and what were the conditions that could keep this museum piece most safe?

"I think, as a doctor, you have to be a little bit more comfortable with risk, because if you don't take risks, no one will ever prescribe anything, or do surgery. You have to know, 'This could go wrong, but I can accept the consequences, and take the calculated, educated risk.' In a job like mine, things aren't that fast moving; it's more about being conservative. There's a reason it's called 'art conservation.' For you, the pleasure to be had by being out in the field outweighs the risk of running into a snake.

"When I grew up in Israel, there were all these phobias that got put in my head. And snakes was one of them. We didn't have rattlesnakes there. I think the ones we had you call 'asps'? They'd tell us, 'Don't stick your hand into a hole. Don't kick a big rock over.' I think I told you about the two boys I used to go out into nature with. When I developed breasts, they wouldn't go out with me anymore – because they didn't want to do that kind of thing with girls. But before that, there was this one time that we saw a snake. I screamed. But one of them had a hoe. And they grabbed it, and chopped the head off. That memory is branded in my head. Sheared there. Is 'sheared' the right word?"

'Seared', I said, feeling relieved I didn't have to spend my life speaking a foreign tongue.

Then, the memory of April suggesting we move to Israel when things were really looking bad for us with FQHC flashed in my head.

"It was the same for my grandparents," she'd said. "When things got so bad for the Jews in Europe, they left Czechoslovakia, to come to this country, where they had no friends, and didn't know the language. But there was no choice, so they came to this foreign land, and learned…"

CHAPTER FORTY-TWO

"I wanted to tell you a story about what happened today with Ini," April said. "Ini crawled under the fence and was playing with Bright Eyes. Then, she got hold of one of Bright Eyes's balls and began guarding it, and went under the table, so she wouldn't play. So I took the ball from her and put it on the table. And I was talking to Ryan. Blah, blah, blah. And I wasn't paying attention. And then, Ini came up, and I was petting her, saying, 'Oh, how nice. How affectionate.' Then, she got up and grabbed the ball in her mouth and went back down.

"And Ryan and I laughed! I was like, 'That was tricky, tricky.' She really thought about that. I know it. She sat thinking, 'How do I get that ball back?' She's like, 'Oh, I'm going to cozy up to mom, make her feel good, and when she isn't paying attention, grab it.' Because I actually didn't notice it – it was Ryan on the other end of the table starting to laugh, or else I wouldn't have even known. She was all cuddly, and I was petting her. She totally worked me."

"Afterwards," she continued, "Ryan and me took the dogs out. As we were walking on the street, some people stopped us and said between Ini and Bright Eyes, it looked like we walking a coyote and a wolf..."

CHAPTER FORTY-THREE

Ini ran ahead into the fields.

"Ini's more delicate than other dogs," April said. "Where other dogs her size, height and length are more bulked up, Ini is slender and elegant... I wouldn't call her 'dainty.' That would imply physically out of step. She's a lot more powerful than dainty. She can jump and run and switch directions in a heartbeat. I would call her graceful and athletic. Like a ballet dancer – capable and powerful in her elegant, slender way."

My thoughts drifted to April's sister, Lea, who had been a ballet dancer until she hurt her leg. In fact, it was Lea who introduced me to April.

"Because she liked the way you danced," April reminded me. "She thought you could be a ballet dancer. And then there's me, and I'm such not... I mean, I am a dancer – just a free-flowing dancer."

Which I prefer, I thought.

"I worry when Ini rumbles roughly with heavier dogs," April continued. "I look at her thin little legs, and I get worried because I don't want her to get hurt. Even though she has a really strong heart and loves to play rough, her body is just more delicate than those other dogs."

I smiled.

"Have to watch out for you, Ini," I said. "Like to rumble with the big dogs."

"Yeah, like her dad," she said. "Except that you take on the big fights – and usually get knocked down. *You* need to watch it!..."

CHAPTER FORTY-FOUR

"Most people are not like you, Michael," she continued. "You would stand by your principles even if they cause harm to you personally. Most people aren't like that. They got their little houses to pay off, and kids to put through college and tuition. Little yards to beautify, and at some point that becomes more important. More realist.

"There definitely are a people like you – they're all over the history books as martyrs, who get clobbered on. Or who moved things – but mostly get clobbered on. That's why they make the news, and the history books. Because most people aren't like them.

"I remember talking with your uncle at the wedding. He said, 'Michael doesn't aim to please. He isn't a people-pleaser.' And some places want you to aim to please. And you can't do it. You just can't do it! It doesn't feel right to you if it's against the health of the patient you're treating. It just doesn't matter what the consequences to yourself, you can't do it.

"And you like it when people like you. You do. You really do. That's the funny part of it. That's the irony. You're really happy when people are happy with you. But you can't do it if you think it's against what's right for either society or that specific person. You really get off on people enjoying you, being grateful to you, appreciating you, liking you. But you're not a slut to it. You don't do whatever is necessary to get that reaction from people."

"Your uncle might be a selfish man," she continued, "but what he said did have a ring of truth to it. I told him, 'No, Mike aims to heal.'"

"And this is beautiful, Mike," she brightened. "That the word has spread by word-of-mouth, and patients are coming to you. And these are not patients who are being thrown at you from within the medical center from other doctors. These are people out there hearing a recommendation to see this new doctor at the clinic who's really good. Who really listens. Who really cares about people.

"And they're coming out to see you. And these are probably people who would avoid seeing somebody as long as they could hold off - until they get to the point where they really have to. And they're picking you to go see. So it's a pat on the back, and not a weight on your shoulders."

"It's because you embody many of their Lakota values. Values which are personality traits Lakota people encourage everyone to want to develop. Generosity. Perseverance – that's a big one, and you got it in spades. Bravery. Honor. You do everything the right way. People trust you."

"And the people here are healing you, too," she continued. "Even the first time you came here, before you were taking care of the people here as a doctor, you were affected by the suicides that happened here. You had that early childhood experience with suicide, so it's a psychic wound you're needing to heal in yourself. I knew it before, but the way you talked about it when that suicide cluster happened on the Reservation that first time you came out here, it illuminated it for me - put a spotlight on it. Illuminated your personal story because of what happened here, and why you got so affected, and became so involved.

"Having listened to your life stories, zooming in on the pivotal moments in your psyche are the early memories of the fights between your dad and your mom; your dad leaving; Chrissie's death; and the accident you had when the car hit you. I think they're all the major events of your childhood that you keep going back to..."

CHAPTER FORTY-FIVE

Passing a couple on the trail, Ini enthusiastically greeted them.

"Ini loves everybody," April said. "And appearances don't matter to her. It's almost as though she's stargazing when she sees people. Any person is like a good friend. Have you noticed that? Even the grumpiest, stenchiest person ever, and she still wants to be good friends with them.

"I think that's how you are. You love everybody. Or, at least, they have worth and value. Not everybody feels that way. I think that's why your patients respond to you the way they do."

April admired the flowering trees. Most were past peak bloom and what remained of their flowers were hid by green leaves.

"Going from sexy trees to working trees," she said. "It's like they make this great hurrah, and then they have to go from putting out all that energy to making energy for the future."

April lagged behind, smelling the budding flowers on the trees. As I moved ahead, Ini stared at me with puffed cheek, as though in disapproval; then, she went running back to April. I'd been continuing forward when Ini came charging towards me, blocking my way till April caught up.

"Did you think daddy was getting too far ahead and he needed to go back?" April said, scratching Ini's forehead. "That's the way I felt when I was so far behind you that I was all by myself. And then Ini would find me, running back-and-forth to where you were, so I wasn't as worried because she was there and she wasn't going to let me get lost. I would be like there by myself and suddenly there was Ini."

"Mommy's protector," she concluded. "It's her herding instinct. She wants us to all stay together. It seems she's accepted me into the pack..."

Passing a family, Ini edged towards the children.

"Ini loves kids," April said. "She would have loved it if we had a child for her to play with."

Bowing my head, I stayed silent.

"That's okay," she said. "You know how people call babies their 'bundle of joy'?... Today, I was calling Ini my 'little bundle of fur'..."

CHAPTER FORTY-SIX

At the house April played ball with Ini; Ini returning each toss by placing the ball on April's lap.

"She's so good, Mike," she said. "You're so lucky to have her."

April caressed her.

"Ini has unusually soft fur," she said. "You did some good praying that day. You got rewarded.

"I think that even though you were praying for me that night Ini showed up, really, she was the answer to your prayers. Right, Ini?"

Ini got on the couch with April.

"And she really did need you," she added. "She was meant to be in the pile of bones at the bottom of the ravine behind the police station where they dumped all the rest of those dogs bodies. She needed you just like you needed her."

Then, she turned.

"Mike, where's your friend Stan?" she asked. "You never talk about him. Have you seen him since you came back?"

Stan was gone. I went to my laptop and pulled up his last email.

I am saddened that I am not there to be with you. Despite all the positive energy, awesome ceremony and people, wonderful memories on the Rez, I had to leave. I have to maintain sufficient income to keep five households running, all filled with loved ones profoundly affected by poverty, etc. Hence I could not simply follow my dream and the line of greatest hope, as so many depended on my every and found work and a steady pay check at Fort Peck.

See, not much help huh. Still, try to generate and reverbate to positive energy.

Your friend,

Stan

"That must have been quite a blow," April said. "The two of you were pretty tight."

I nodded. A year ago he'd been the first person I'd met here; following the suicide cluster, he'd introduced me to native ways, healing ceremonies, Medicine men, educators, artists; he'd offered his friendship, and opened a window to his world; now, his restaurant and Lakota Youth Center were closed, and my prospects as a physician, markedly different.

April looked away, her expression changed and features darkened.

"I really hate those people at FQHC," she said. "I try not to be sad and accept it. But it was our chance to have a child, and it was taken away from us. Why do you think that Dr. Lang turned on you that way? Didn't you like him? And the two of you would talk about baseball and blah-blah-blah?... When you were under Jessica's auspices, he was friendly with you. But the moment that Jessica's protection from Administration disappeared, he did whatever he had to survive. He turned on you.

"Jessica was a special person. Either she was able to interact with Administration in a way that you weren't being bullied, or she wanted to protect people, so she would do things that turned out well. I bet wherever Jessica is, people are happy. I bet she creates the healthiest work environment in whatever organization she's in. She was like you – she was a NHSC scholar, and had to be there for three years? She probably didn't like the organization at FQHC. She probably didn't like what they were doing. She was gonna leave there just as soon as she was able. And I bet where she went to is a pretty decent place to work. I bet you she's a pretty good judge of character, and she was doing as much interviewing of them, as they were interviewing her."

She sighed.

"The reason that FQHC did what they did was because they didn't have a case," she continued. "If it had ever been brought to a hearing or a courtroom, they would've had no chance – especially since this was an NHSC scholar that they took in.

"But you didn't have a leg to stand on because it was an 'at will' contract. So, they could let you go at will. But where they were sneaky and underhanded and evil was when they tried to make it into a competence issue. They did it to try to get you to leave quietly on your own. Because if talk of you being incompetent ever came out, it would affect your ability to get hired anywhere. I mean, if you're looking at an applicant who has an employer who says the reason they let you go was because you were incompetent, are you going to really listen to what that person is going to say? Are you going to look at the cases yourself? Are you going to want to spend your time doing that? You have your own work to do. Are you going to hire this person? You're not going to hire him. Just malicious rumors can ruin you. Because people are going to assume that the organization performed its due diligence. People are going to assume that nobody wants to fire and they're not going to say it if they didn't believe it. Not every place is run like the government, where they have to prove you're incompetent."

She shook her head.

"FQHC was a joke," she said. "They market themselves as a fighter for the rights of the underserved and underprivileged, but what they turned out to be was a persecutor of docs who wouldn't give out pain medications."

She shook her head.

"They went after you when we were just married," she said. "And my grandmother had just died. And they knew it! They knew it. That CEO actually sent you a condolence letter after grandma died. And two weeks after us getting married. A week later, they slammed you with this stuff. Awful people.

"My biological clock was ticking. If they hadn't messed you up then, we would have started right away – at the moment I was ovulating. We probably would've had a kid. That's why I'm so mad at that organization. I hate them. I hate them more than I hate anybody in the world – except for the Nazis. They seriously took away our chance of having a child.

"They hurt me. You know me – I don't wish harm on anybody. If I see somebody hurt on the side of the road, I go and I help. If I see that CEO on the side of the road – deathly injured, about to die – I'd probably walk on by. The way this happened, I'd probably just walk on by and laugh in his face.

"He hurt me. Ruthless son of a bitch. He ran that place with intimidation. He was a bully. I could see that – When we walked into that office that first day, and you were giving them some papers, and I turned around and asked if you really wanted to work here? It were like, you walked in there, and I could feel it – It was being run by an evil son-of-a-bitch. And he's still there. Evil son-of-a-bitch. And I don't talk about people like that. I hate that person. I really hate that person. Really hate."

"But I think after this, they'll leave you alone," resuming a subdued tone. "They don't want it dug into. They'll say you resigned, and there's nothing in your file. You just have to finish your NHSC obligation,   then   you   can   come   home..."

CHAPTER FORTY-SEVEN

April asked about things at the hospital? I said work was tense. On-call every night. Sick patients. I thought it was all leaving me quick to anger.

"The odd thing, though," I said, "I'm not that way with Ini."

"I think she changes your mood," April said. "It's like you go out with her on a walk and you come back more relaxed and happier. Dogs are well known for being companion animals. I think she gives you a shot of oxytocin, so that you get that in the brain."

"Ini's in your endorphin system," she asserted. "I think that I was once in your endorphin system, too, but, of late, you plucked me out. Some people, you spend a lot of time trying to take them out of your endorphin system, but others, even after a lifetime of trying, you don't succeed."

She looked away.

"After over ten years of being apart, you came looking for me," she said. "I think the way our relationship ended all those years ago, you never had the chance to pluck me out. Now, maybe you have?..."

When we got together,
I fell so head over heels in love with you.
I bonded to you.
Before that, I would be happy meeting people,
But there was a place inside always seeking to be filled
And was empty
And you filled that place.
I connected to you
on a really deep heart and soul level.
Now, I wonder,
Is there a way?
I know we've gone through some difficult times.
I'm left wondering, Can we go back to that place?
Because I want to.
I really do.
I really want to try.
I have moments
where I am so in love
and connected to you –
When I'm so amazed at the things you do
and the person who you are,
and the things you think.
And then I have other moments...
I don't know –
I want to always be in love with you.
But maybe that's not realistic.

CHAPTER FORTY-EIGHT

Sitting alone among April's sketches and writings, a knock came from the door. It was Somay. Opening the door, I led her into the darkened room with no thought of switching on another light or turning down the music coming from the CD player.

I'm so glad that you came
I'm so glad you remembered
To see how it ends
Our last Dance together.

"What are you listening to?" she asked.
The Cure, I responded. Tears in Rain.
"It sounds depressing," she said. "Is it because your wife left?"
I nodded.
"Does it make you sad that you aren't with her?"
That's part of it, I said.
Then, I recalled times I'd heard those words before and fell silent...

CHAPTER FORTY-NINE

The first storm of the season was approaching and my supervisor, Dr. James Curtiz, pulled me aside.

"We're going to close the clinic for rest of the day," he said, "due to the severe weather we're expecting...."

Walking home against the strong winds and swirling snow, I looked out at the dark blue horizon and thought about the stories of Crazy Horse – ancestor to these people, who'd lived only about a hundred years ago, and, as well as a great warrior, is remembered for going out into a blizzard to hunt, so his people wouldn't starve.

Once home I called to Ini. Despite the sheets of falling snow and harsh billowing wind, she trotted through the door without hesitation.

Arriving at Somay's I asked if she and Wesley would like to join Ini and me for a walk?

"I don't think it's a good time to be out, Dr. Mike," she said. "It's supposed to be a bad storm."

Undeterred, I continued our trek into the storm. There wasn't a blizzard that Ini wouldn't follow me into and I loved that about my companion.

Ascending a hill Ini ran ahead. As she sniffed along the periphery of a tree, I noted some movement of the branches. Suddenly, three large bucks tore out, Ini chasing after them in head-long pursuit. The bucks were each much larger than Ini and it struck me that a single kick from any of them could kill her (as she was right at their heels). Still, I couldn't help but feel a certain admiration: There was Ini obeying her instinct, running full-bore ahead without fear or thought for the repercussions and peril it might entail.

"Ini!" I called. "Ini!"

But it was to no avail – the four of them disappearing over the top of the ridge. Above me were two hawks; in the swirling snow, they flew in and out of sight, disappearing into the nebulous borders of the grey storm clouds. Whisks of snow leapt from the ground; I hoped that it might be Ini dashing back to me, but was only the dance of whirlwinds. Ini was still nowhere in sight, and the freezing wind that permeated my clothes was so cold my hands ached.

"Ini! Ini!"

I strained to listen for her, but there was only the sound of the billowing wind. The only other sound was the calls from a crow, as it flipped in the wind. I looked for tracks, and seemed to find some; maybe, Ini's. Maybe, the deer. I couldn't be sure.

Then, my phone rang; I recognized Somay's number.

"The storm radio just went off," she said. "It says the blizzard is getting worse. In a little while, there's going to be complete white-out. You can get really disoriented in white out. Are you and Ini back home?"

No, I said. I've lost her. I've been looking for her, but can't find her.

"You need to go home, Dr. Mike," she insisted. "The dog knows the area. She's alright. She'll come home. Dogs can survive those temperatures. You have to be concerned about yourself now. In a little while, you'll have no way of knowing where you are…"

I walked down until I had a view of the community below; but the closer I got, the more anxiety I experienced.

Had one of those deer injured Ini? I thought. Was she lying out in the snow somewhere unconscious? Had she re-broken her leg?

I ventured back to the hills. But turning to look back, I found that I could no longer see the town. Trying to find my way, I stumbled and went sliding down the ravine, the only thing halting my descent was a young slender tree, which, by my latching on to, snapped in two. Staring at it, I caught my breath; I thought how (because of me) it would never grow to maturity. It had given its life, so I might live. Using it as a staff now, I pulled myself out of the ravine. I would have liked to keep it, but given the freezing wind, there was no holding it; I had to keep my hands by my core to keep them warm. I planted it into the ground and moved on.

Removing my gloves, my hands were beet red and swollen, like they belonged on a stuffed dummy; I was unable to close them into a fist, and they seemed to flop, like I wasn't in control of them.

Just then, Ini appeared at my side. Ears down, snow coated her fur; her lashes were frozen along the contours of her eyes, so she had to squint; and icicles ran along the groove left by the surgical scar on her leg. Otherwise, she was unharmed.

God be merciful, I thought.

"Ini, let's go home..."

CHAPTER FIFTY

The thick, swirling sheets of snow made it nearly impossible to see, and felt like tiny daggers slicing at my eyes. Ini trailed behind me, her ears set low. Not knowing where to go, I stood planted, my thoughts wandering to happenings on the Rez.

What if in one of those overcrowded homes, someone says the wrong thing, or makes a wrong move, and there's an argument, and someone feels like he or she has to get out? I thought. Or, worse, they're pushed out? What would they do then? How would that person survive?

I felt the urge to run to them – find them – say something to keep them safe – Keep them alive through the storm.

I couldn't see anything in front of me, and my leg was going into spasm. Ini was still just behind me; I could still see her through the blowing snow.

You and me, Ini, I thought. We need to stay together. That you don't like it, I won't apply ischemic compressions on your leg anymore. Of course, you couldn't understand why I was doing it. You thought I was just causing you pain. From now on, Somay would just do it on me alone. As I heal, you heal. Just stay with me. Stay with me.

Then, in the distance, something seemed to be taking shape; an upright figure that looked like a cross between the abominable snowman and the Michelin man; coming towards us; then waved and called out with a woman's voice.

"Dr. Mike. Dr. Mike."

I stood staring. It didn't make sense. Was I losing it? Had I finally passed over to my mother's illness?

"Dr. Mike."

It was Somay – gowned in what I imagined was every article of clothing she owned.

"I got all geared up figuring that I had to go out into the blizzard to locate you and Ini," she said. "I got into all my snow gear to go looking for you."

Through countless snow drifts, Somay led Ini and me back to her home. I tried to talk but could hardly move my jaws, so what did come out left me sounding drunk.

Inside, it felt like I was still stumbling around and could barely use my hands. Removing the gloves, my hands were near white.

Somay filled the bathroom sink with warm water and led me there to soak them. Gazing in the mirror, I looked like something out of Dr. Zhivago; ice around my nose and eyes, my skin felt firm and waxy. In the other room Somay was crouched and delivering a firm but good-natured scolding to Ini.

"Ini, you're supposed to protect Dr. Mike," she said. "Not run off, so he should search aimlessly for you in the middle of a blizzard..."

CHAPTER FIFTY-ONE

By morning the storm had mostly lifted and the sun could be made out through the clouds in the horizon. Returning home, Ini ran to Bright Eyes, who was outside with another dog that I surmised from its gangly limbs and awkward movements was a large puppy.

"My daughter begged me to let her bring it home last night," Ryan said. "The mother was a stray, and three other puppies in the litter died during the storm... They froze to death... Yeah, the mother couldn't take care of them..."

Arriving at the hospital I joined the others in the conference room for Morning Report. Dr. Curtiz wore a somber expression.

"Tom Eagle died of hypothermia yesterday," he said.

I looked up. Tom was a local artist. I'd purchased some of his art; he'd recently repaired the small dreamcatcher that hung from my rearview mirror.

"He'd been trying to get home when the blizzard hit," Curtiz continued. "He got caught in the white out and his car slipped off the road into a ditch. He'd called his wife; she told him to stay in the car until help arrived, but he insisted on going, saying he knew the way home. She contacted family, friends, the police - they all went looking for him. They didn't find him, though; not until the storm broke. He was about a couple miles from his car. Worst of all, he'd been so completely turned around that he'd been going the opposite direction of where he lived, and froze to death miles from his home."

I bowed my head.

That could have been me and Ini, I thought, had Somay not come and found us.

"Tom had been in my office a week ago," Curtiz said. "He came to sell his art. We talked about the hospital commissioning him to paint a mural for the entrance."

I remembered that day; I'd seen Tom leaving the office, calling back to Curtiz with enthusiasm for the planned project.

"I bought a couple pieces of his art that day," Curtiz continued. "They're right in my office, hanging on the wall…"

Attending Tom's wake I could hardly believe the man in the casket was the same man I knew. Rather than the proud artist of a week ago who'd walked out of Dr. Curtiz's office with his chest puffed up and hardy voice, he literally looked deflated, his body thin, like a mummified relic from a time long ago.

He'd been so alive, I thought. So utterly full of life.

Orville stood next to me.

"The last time I saw Tom," he said, "he was talking about a course he was going to teach at the community college. I swear it's getting more and more like our people are here one day and gone the next…"

CHAPTER FIFTY-TWO

Somay came to the house accompanied by a small boy.

"This is my nephew, Wesley," she said. "Wesley, say hi to Dr. Mike."

Unsmiling, Wesley extended his hand and gave me a firm shake in the traditional native way. He was maybe five years old. Ini came out wagging her whole body, obviously interested in Wesley. But Wesley wanted nothing to do with her, and the firm way that Wesley pushed Ini away left me struck by the seeming fearlessness and strength of the little boy.

"Wesley has grown up with horses his whole life," Somay told me. "He knows what it is to hold his own with something twenty times his size."

Ini excitedly ran to Somay now.

"Hi Ini!" she said, as she kneeled to greet her, Ini's paws on Somay's shoulders. Wesley looked on with bored expression.

"Why don't we all go for a walk?" Somay said.

Making our way towards the badlands behind the house, Wesley trailed behind.

"I'm sorry about Wesley," she said. "His father died not long ago, and, since then, my sister's had a hard time with him. I think it's because Wesley feels – with his father gone – that it's his responsibility to assume the role of man of the house. I think it's just his way of coping."

"How did his father die?" I asked.

"Cory was a bronc rider," she said. "He broke his neck when he was stumped on by a bull. It left him a quad. After that, he kept on getting sicker, until his body finally gave out.

"Wesley was just a baby when the accident happened, and only knew Cory as a quad. I think that's where he got the feeling like he had to be the man of the house. Five years old, but that's the way he sees things - like he has to take care of all of us. Dad tries to help, but Wesley is very strong..."

CHAPTER FIFTY-THREE

Somay announced that she and Wesley were going to see a movie in town.

"Dad's going to meet us," she said. "Are you sure you don't want to come with us, Dr. Mike?"

But recalling the veterinarian's admonition about town gossip, I declined.

Somay and Wesley had hardly stepped through the door before I stood regretting my decision. Then, I heard a familiar sounding thump – like when a person takes a fall – and Wesley calling out.

"Dr. Mike, come quick!" he said. "Aunt Somay hit her head."

Somay lay on the street, whimpering, and moving her hand to the back of her head.

"I must have slipped," she said. "Am I bleeding?... My head really hurts."

Somay's speech was slow and partly slurred; I thought she might have suffered a concussion and suggested we call an ambulance.

"No, I don't want to go to the hospital," she said. "Maybe I could just lie down."

Assisting her, I guided her into the house.

"I better call dad," she said. "He was expecting to meet us at the theater..."

Orville arrived a short time later.

"What happened?" he asked.

"She slipped and must have hit her head on the curb," I said. "I wanted to take her to the emergency room, but she wouldn't go."

"She doesn't trust the hospital," he said. "It goes way back... Her aunt was sterilized there... She went to have her baby, and after the birth, they did a tubal ligation on her without her consent. They used to do that kind of thing to the women back then. I don't think they do it anymore... That happened when Somay was about six, but she's never forgotten. Even my daughter-in-law – Wesley's mom – refused to go to the hospital to have Wesley... Wesley was born the traditional way; when she was ready to give birth, she selected a woman to help her, and had him in the house. And after he was born, that woman took him and uttered a special prayer, then smudged the house with sage..."

CHAPTER FIFTY-FOUR

"Can I have something for my eyes?" Somay asked. "The light is hurting them."

I took a bandana from the dresser, and placed it around her head.

"I think I might have used the same bandana on April," I said, "when her eyes hurt… She had meningitis… It happened during our first year together. She had headache and neck pain and light-sensitivity, and I told her I thought she needed to go to the hospital for a lumbar puncture. She asked if I could do it? I'd performed lots of them during my residency, but wasn't credentialed at any of the hospitals, so there was no way I could do it. She asked if I really thought she needed one? I said, really, I thought she had a viral meningitis, and since there was really no treatment for it except supportive care, it probably wouldn't make much difference in how she was treated. In the end we decided I would observe her, and take her to the hospital if she got worse.

"It was kind of sweet. She'd be wearing that bandana because her eyes hurt, and I'd lead her to the bathroom, or to the kitchen to eat. One day her father called, just to ask how things were going. When I told him I thought April had meningitis but was getting better, he got really upset. Later, when her family found out, some were really upset. 'April has meningitis and you didn't take her to the hospital!' It turns out that April had a cousin who'd died of meningitis, so I could understand why he was so alarmed."

I looked up at Orville.

"Now, I'm going to get in trouble with your father for not taking you to the hospital," I said.

Orville chuckled, but Somay's expression was unchanged.

105

"When April had meningitis," I continued, "she'd say it hurt to think."

The howl of the wind could be heard through the walls, and I looked out the window; it appeared another blizzard was beginning to rage.

What am I doing talking about April? I thought. Like Somay wants to hear about someone else's suffering right now?

"I had meningitis," Somay said. "It did hurt to think…"

CHAPTER FIFTY-FIVE

Standing over the sink I warmed a towel to place over Somay's head; Orville stood nearby.

"Orville, I'm sorry for what happened to your daughter," I said. "If I'd just accepted her invitation to join you at the movies, probably none of this would have happened."

Orville stood quiet.

"In our tradition," he began, "there are three ways you become a member of the family. One, you have to be the same bloodline. Two, you become a member through marriage. The third way is by adoption. Sometimes, they call it, 'Hunka' - that's a very important ceremony. When you become a member of the family by adoption, you become a full member of that family. That whole family will accept you. You might befriend somebody. You might become very close. The two of you can share and keep confidential things for each other. Somebody who you can honestly share things with, and not be afraid it will be talked about. Someone you can trust. And somebody who you can take care of if anything happens to that person - You have the ability to take care of them. And that somebody feels the same way about you. Sometimes, this happens between a man and a woman. They become very close. There is no romance. It is just like finding a sister or brother that you share. Some people think you're like that because you want something, but that's not the case. I think it's that way with you and my daughter..."

CHAPTER FIFTY-SIX

"Relationships are so important among our people," Orville continued. "We always look after our people and relatives. It's very confusing sometimes in the modern world. One time, there was a medicine man from here who was invited to Washington, DC. Some church leaders invited him to come for a conference. He said to me, 'Come with me and translate for me.' So I went with him.

"It was a four-day conference. And, one day, we had some time, so we went into town and walked around, and we went to the Washington Monument. But, on the way, we went through some places where there were street people. They were sleeping on those grills over the sewers. They had their little shelters. They walked around with carts with all their belongings. So, he was really watching.

"Well, we got to the Washington Monument, and somehow we climbed to the top. We had a good tour. Then, we came down. We were sitting out there, and he's watching these people, pushing their carts from trash can to trash can, looking for food to eat. He sat there watching it, and said, 'Don't they at least have one relative?' I said, 'I'm sure they do. But this is how it is out here. You look after yourself and that's it.' Boy, he couldn't believe that. We came home to the reservation, and we had a ceremony, and he told the people - he said, 'You don't know how lucky you are - That you don't live in the   city   -   *where   nobody   cares...*'"

CHAPTER FIFTY-SEVEN

"I feel dizzy," Somay said, "and my neck is bothering me."

The muscles of her neck felt tight.

"I had to have surgery there a few years ago," she responded. "They put me on all kinds of pain medicine. Finally, I told them I didn't want any. I wonder if the kind of thing you do with Ini would help?"

Applying pressure, she winced.

"Ouch!" she said. "That's really tender."

"Do you want me to stop?" I asked

"No, I think it's helping," she said.

But despite Somay's entreaty, Ini was visibly agitated, and jumped on the couch, and got in between us, inserting her muzzle under my arm, and nudging my hand away.

"I think Ini knows what you're going through," I said.

Somay reached out and pulled Ini close.

"I   love   you,   Ini,"   she   said...

CHAPTER FIFTY-EIGHT

As I worked the muscles of Somay's neck, a memory surfaced.

"It's funny the things you think of," I said. "When I was young, my mother told me about falling from a tree. It happened in some fields just beyond her home in Far Rockaway. She loved to climb and referred to herself a 'tomboy.'

"So, she was climbing this tree and the branch broke off. And when she fell, there was some glass underneath – like maybe a broken *Coca-Cola* bottle - and she cut her head. She started to cry; and it was raining; and she said it felt like the tears were rolling back in her head; and the rain was going under her clothes, but instead of cold, it felt warm. Naturally, it was blood she was the feeling, coming from the wound."

"How old was she?" Somay asked.

I didn't know. She'd told me my Uncle hadn't been born yet; since he was twelve years younger, she was maybe ten.

"She said she ran home," I continued, "but her mother wasn't there (She was out playing cards). Fortunately, the maid was present, and put a towel to my mother's head.

"She said her mother (my grandma) showed up about the same time as the doctor; she remembered her mother standing in the doorway.

"The doctor stitched the wound, but only used four stitches, so it left quite a scar. The hair never grew back over it. When she showed me, it looked like a lightning bolt running all through her hairlines.

"She said they called her 'brave', because the doctor didn't use anesthesia. A few days later they got her a feather to put in her hair, like an 'Indian brave.'"

Looking at Somay, we exchanged smiles.

"My wife grew up in Israel," I continued. "But even there she had a feeling for native peoples. One of my favorite pictures is her as a kid, sitting on a tree branch wearing war paint, a feather in her hair."

"That's cute," Somay said. "Was she wearing one of those bands around her head?... Oh, I like your wife, Dr. Mike. I hope I get to meet her one day..."

CHAPTER FIFTY-NINE

Somay asked Orville to take her and Wesley home. Afterwards, I drove into town to wash my clothes at the laundromat. Inside, there was a young native woman and a little girl. The woman had dyed blond hair with pink streaks; the girl seemed spirited, eager to help. I wonder how they were related? Was the young woman the girl's mother? Or an older sister? I didn't know.

An overhead television was playing a broadcast of *60 minutes;* the first installment featured a female executive with a six figure income; she was talking about being offered a high position in a rival firm; she said she wanted to accept the job, but held out for more money. I gazed at the little girl; she was sitting on a rocking horse coin ride that didn't work; bouncing as though imagining she was riding; and I wondered that she'd ever be offered a six-figure income?

Folding my clothes, I continued to ponder the fairness of it all; I wanted to ask the woman if I might perhaps pay the little girl to help me, so I might talk with her, listen to her, find out what she aspired to, and what inspired her?

Just then, a young man entered the laundromat. He was white and rugged looking, and walked directly to the young woman and began talking with her; the little girl, meanwhile, stayed back, appearing wary.

The young man went to his car. By this time I was done with my laundry. Making my way out, I held the door for the young man as he came back in; he didn't acknowledge me, and wore a cold expression as he walked past. Looking back through the glass, he was lifting the woman into the air; the little girl standing nearby, appearing lost and unsure...

CHAPTER SIXTY

In the morning I checked on Somay.

"I'm feeling better," she said.

She suggested we find Wesley and take a walk.

"Are you sure you're up to it?" I asked. "It looks like it might snow."

"I like the snow," she said.

Wesley was feeding the horses, stuffing hay through the stables, and filling the troughs with water. Defiant at first, he refused Somay's entreaties to join us; then, after we walked away, he called after us. Running towards us – standing tall with outward chest – he displayed a powerful energy. Ini ran to fetch him, then galloped alongside Wesley. Wesley was winded when he caught up with us, and hunkered with his hands to his thighs. Ini took several mouthfuls of snow; when she looked up, her nose was covered. Wesley smiled; his features relaxed, it was like seeing him as a little boy for the first time.

"Your dog eats snow," he said.

Somay smiled.

"Yum," she said. "Cold snow cone. Ini sure loves her snow. It's probably what she ate when her mother weaned her from her milk – like when you have a craving for something you ate when you were a kid."

Considering the season when I found her, I wondered that snow was the only thing that Ini had to drink?

"Was Ini super hungry that evening you brought her home from the sweat lodge?" Wesley asked.

I didn't recall. Indeed, Ini was something of a picky eater.

"She's not picky about snow," Somay said. "The snow cone she ate had a lot of sand in it. Those were some gritty, sandy snow cones."

Just as long as there wasn't any yellow snow in it, I commented. Wesley laughed.

"'Yellow snow,'" he repeated, giggling.

Approaching the river, snow began falling, and the wind picked up. Ini ran ahead.

"Look how beautiful the snow is recording Ini paw prints," Somay said.

Up ahead, Ini was digging. When she lifted her head, she had a large bone in her mouth.

"Probably belonged to a buffalo," Somay said.

Ini hunkered in the snow and gnawed at the bone, licking the marrow. Fearing it might cause food poisoning, I took it away from her, and flung it in the river. Ini became agitated; she jumped, and then pulled and tugged at my heel with a ferocity I found unnerving. I wondered that, in taking her spoils, I'd triggered a primal response? Her leaping, darting movements were so quick as to transform her into a blur before my eyes. She bit into my boots, and thrashed at them till ripping the fabric. Then, she growled, and it felt like our usual circling game had changed from one of play to that of predator and prey? Like a wolf tearing at its victim's ankle.

Turning in the blowing snow, I looked out at Somay and Wesley; it was as though viewing them through a strobe light; them moving in slow motion; laughing, amused by the spectacle; to them it was still a game; they didn't understand that Ini was behaving different than I'd ever seen her.

I didn't want to risk making the situation worse by scolding Ini; given her current state, I wasn't sure how she'd respond. I'd never sought to particularly train her; she'd come to me a feral creature of the wild, and I'd tried to respect that. But, in the process, had I made myself vulnerable? Had I put myself in harm's way?...

CHAPTER SIXTY-ONE

Just then, Somay snatched Ini, embracing her and stroking her head.

"Sweet girl," she said. "Sweet girl."

Looking on, I was concerned that Ini might turn and bite Somay. I'd been unsuspectedly bitten that way when I'd been Wesley's age; I'd been petting a dog that belonged to my father's friend, Jim, when it lunged and nearly ripped off my ear. On the operating table the physician who stitched me joked, "We're you going to send your ear to a girlfriend, like Vincent van Gogh?"

"What happened with the dog that bit you?" Somay asked.

Nothing at the time. Returning from the Emergency Room, my father and Jim asked what I'd done to provoke the animal? I said I didn't know – that I'd simply been petting it. They'd looked at me, doubtful. A month later, though, the dog bit the face of Jim's newborn son; Jim took the dog to the top of a hill, and shot it.

Somay turned, then sang softly in Lakota in Ini's ear. Ini looked on with interest.

"I think she likes it," she said, smiling. "She wags her tail when I sing it to her."

Then, Ini pranced and danced about in the snow.

What are you singing? I asked.

"'A heart full of love,'" she responded. "Do you think that's a good   song   for   Ini?..."

CHAPTER SIXTY-TWO

Making our way back Wesley appeared tired and lagged behind. "Could I ride on your back, Dr. Mike?" he asked.

Hoisting Wesley on my back, Ini looked at us perturbed, as though bothered by the two of us having seemingly merged into one new creature and offered a chorus of uncharacteristic, high-pitched howls. As she nipped at the heels of my boots, I chased after her, neighing like a horse and bucking and galloping, as Wesley laughed uncontrollably.

"Do you have any friends, Dr. Mike?" he asked. "I'm probably the first buddy you've made out here. It's good to have a buddy. Someone who you could talk to and do things with…"

In the distance I made out a pick-up truck parked next to the stables and the outlines of a tall, slightly bent, broad-shouldered man wearing a cowboy hat.

"Grandpa!" Wesley called out.

Wesley jumped down from my back and ran to Orville; he was still talking about our adventures when Somay and I reached them.

"And Ini eats snow, Grandpa!" Wesley said. "It's probably something she learned as a pup before Dr. Mike found her."

Somay's expression changed, and she took a couple steps back.

"Something the matter?" I asked.

"And Dr. Mike said, 'I hope Ini doesn't eat any yellow snow,'" Wesley continued, laughing.

"No, it's not that," Somay told me. "It's just… It's been so long since I've seen Wesley this excited. Like he could be a little boy, and not feel like he had to take care of all of us. Not since my brother…"

Her chin began to quiver, and she covered her mouth.

"I'm   sorry,"   she   said…

CHAPTER SIXTY-THREE

Neither wolf nor dog.
~ Chief Sitting Bull

"I talked to dad about Ini biting at your ankle yesterday," Somay said. "He said Ini might be part wolf. Dad said he had a dog that was part wolf and that's what he would do. He would do it to the other dogs. He said even with the bigger dogs, this one would do it. He said when this dog would do it to the pitbull, the pitbull would drop to one side and lay down. Just go down. I told him, 'Dad, I didn't even know that.' He said, 'Oh, yeah, he controlled them that way, and that's what a wolf does, too.' He said a wolf does it to maim and bring down prey, or to control other wolves in the pack. It's their instinct. When they play, they will go grab at the ankles to get the other one down. It's also the hunting instinct, where if you bite and cut the tendon, it will drop the animal.

"Dad said his dog wouldn't do it to him... Bite at his ankles. But he thought you have a different relationship with Ini than he has with any of his dogs."

I looked off. So was it control or play? Or was I prey to Ini?

"I think it was just her playing with you," Somay said. "Because if she really wanted to hurt you, she would have bit you pretty good."

I recalled the mental image of throwing that bone away just before she started biting at me. Had it been her way of taking out her aggressions?

"She was just letting you know," Somay said. "It was her way of standing her ground. But it is different from what other dogs will do. For a dog, if you don't let a dog do something, or if you're not giving it attention, it will let you know by taking its paw and scratching you.

Dad had a dog that if you didn't pet her or if you play with another dog and not her, she'd come at you and take her paw and swipe you. And that's a control – because she knows she'll get more attention by scratching you. I'd tell her, 'No, no,' and slap her paw down, saying, 'No, you're not going to scratch me.' One time, though, she got me good."

She pulled up her pant leg.

"You see that scar there?" she said. "That's what she did. It was right after she had a litter of nine pups. I was sitting down playing with her puppies and she really got me."

The scar was nearly six inches long, and viewing it, I remembered the time I'd been bitten by a dog.

"But it was my fault," Somay insisted, "because I wasn't paying attention. It was the same thing with Ini the other day. She was just letting you know."

I felt at the scar on my ear, and wondered that (had Ini done something like that to me) if I'd be as charitable?

Somay readjusted her pant leg and petted Ini.

"You bit Dr. Mike because you're part wolf," she said. "You wanted to let him know, didn't you? You were telling him, 'I'm not just a dog – I'm part wolf.'…"

CHAPTER SIXTY-FOUR

Outside I noticed Somay's car wasn't in the driveway.

"I had to take it in for repairs," she said. "The mechanic called about an hour ago and said that they were done. I'm just waiting for dad to get home, so I can pick it up."

I offered to drive her. At the service station, though, the mechanic informed Somay that the car needed additional repairs.

"We found some more problems in the gear shaft," the mechanic said. "We can get back to it in about an hour, if you're willing to wait that long for it."

The mechanic methodically wrote out a new service slip.

"You're Orville's daughter, aren't you?" he said. "I heard your dad talk at the school about what happened to your people and all that. I work at the school, too... I'm a home father at the Sunday school. When I'd talk to the Indian kids and they'd say that they're in the position they're in because of the 'white man,' and how the white man stole their land, you know what I say? I tell them, 'Okay, tell you what – We'll bring some bulldozers out to the Rez, knock down all your homes, take away all your plates, spoons, knives, forks, cups, glasses, tables, stove pots, then we'll leave you with some tents and bring in some buffalo – how's that?' And you know what? They don't want that. They'd rather keep what they have."

"And you know what else?" he added, smiling. "If the white man hadn't come here, you'd still be hunting the buffalo. There'd be no progress."

"My great grandfather used to kill Indians," he continued. "In the winters when the river would freeze over, they'd come over from the other side to our ranch. He'd let the slaughter a cow or two, and bring it back to their starving people. But when they'd get to greedy, he'd shoot'em down, tie them to their horses, slap those horses on the backside, and send them back to where they came from…"

CHAPTER SIXTY-FIVE

Leaving the repair shop Somay was silent. I suggested lunch at the restaurant across the street. On the table were crayons and doodle placemats. Turning the placemat over, I lifted a crayon.

"Care to humor me?" I said.

I sketched her portrait. Smiling eyes, high cheekbones. Somay seemed at ease till a man at another table gestured in my direction.

"Look at the 4-year-old," he said.

Somay recoiled, though I continued drawing.

"Some might interpret your drawing as a cry for help," she said.

"'Cry for help'?" I repeated, nodding. "Yes, I'm crying for help. I'm here in a town where there are those who brag about the baseness of their forefathers – to the very descendants of those they displaced."

Striking the crayon to the paper now, I made fine lines for her long, dark hair.

"So, yes," I said. "I'm crying for help. At the very least, I'm crying for a different reality to escape to. One in which I might imagine – and perhaps capture – a little beauty and fairness and justice in the world."

I shook my head. How could that mechanic have said those things? Even if they were factually correct, had he no decency or sense of decorum?

"Don't worry about it, Dr. Mike," she said. "I've heard it my whole life. I'm used to it. It doesn't bother me."

I depressed the corners of my lips and nodded.

"Well, I'm not used to it," I responded. "It bothered me..."

CHAPTER SIXTY-SIX

Leaving the restaurant Somay said she wanted to visit the bookstore across from the street. Waiting outside I sat on a park bench in the town square and read a newspaper.

"Do you need some tools?"

Looking up from the paper, a native woman stood holding a pair of pliers and a screwdriver.

No, thank you, I said. I have my own.

She appeared somewhat unsteady.

"Well, do you need something else?" she asked.

I narrowed my gaze and stared at her blankly...

About an hour later Somay and I returned to the repair shop.

"We're still not done with the repairs to your vehicle," the manager said. "We're closed tomorrow, so we won't be able to get back to it till Monday."

A burley-looking man swung open the door and approached the counter.

"Tim, how much longer on the repairs to my truck?" he asked.

"Still, not done yet," the manager responded. "Probably won't be too much longer, though."

"I can't wait," the man said, and motioned to a white van parked in front of the station.

Looking at the van, I noticed someone in the backseat appearing to be sleeping. Then, I recognized it was the woman from the town square.

Turning, my eyes met those of the burley fella, who looked back at me with vacant grin...

CHAPTER SIXTY-SEVEN

Sunday I was going to the laundromat. Somay's car was still in the shop, so I called and asked if she needed anything in town?

"I should do a load, too," she said. "Give me a second to get my things..."

Arriving at the laundromat I was surprised to find it empty.

"Everyone's home watching the Academy Awards," Somay said.

"Do you want to watch them?" I asked. "Maybe, they have it playing at the hotel?..."

In the hotel lobby a small group was gathered around the TV watching the Awards. Somay and I joined them. They were friendly, talking and laughing and engaging us in conversation.

"Hey, what about the two of you pulling up a chair and joining the rest of us?" said an older gentleman said.

Just then, the hotel manager appeared and glared at Somay and me.

"Now, everyone here is a guest of the hotel, right?" he said.

I looked at Somay, resignedly. But just as we were about to depart, the older man intervened.

"Yeah, we're all in the wedding party," he told the manager. "We're all guests of the hotel."

Though still looking at Somay and me, the manager now appeared unsure. A moment later he turned and walked off.

The older man smiled, appearing quite pleased. Then, he turned to Somay and me.

"Now what were we talking about?" he said...

CHAPTER SIXTY-EIGHT

After the Awards, Somay and I were making our way to the exit, when we were intercepted by a tipsy young woman in a pink dress and high-heels.

"Hey, would the two of you like to dance with the rest of us?" she asked.

I looked to Somay.

"We won't bite," the young woman added.

I shrugged.

Sure, I said.

"Then, com' on," the woman responded, spiritedly.

She said she was one of the bridesmaids for a wedding held earlier in the day, and led us to a large ballroom. Music blared from amplifiers, and red disco lights illuminated the surroundings; couples danced on the hardwood floor, while others conversed along the sides. Somay and I crossed over to the bar. Standing nearby was a sturdy-looking, Native American fellow.

"I'm the bride's father," he said. "I'm not actually from here. I was born in Sisseton, but taken away from my family and put in foster care when I was just a baby. I had the good fortune of growing up with very caring parents, but every day I had to fight with the kids in school because I was native. I learned to be mean and to fight - skills I took with me into the military. Now, I'm looking to find my way back to my native ways, though I mostly regard myself as a Christian. In the church they teach you praying to anything but Jesus is praying to Satan in the form of evil spirits, and that makes it difficult."

He looked at me, inquisitively.

"Are you Jewish?" he said. "I ask because you look like a Jewish friend I had. I think the same thing that happened to my people as what happened to the Jews at the hands of Hitler and the Nazis. It's exactly the same. We were herded by the government into camps, our children taken away from us by the government, and sent away to places where they were abused and many died. It's the exact same thing..."

CHAPTER SIXTY-NINE

Across the dancefloor, the bride waved to her father.

"It looks like I'm being summoned," he said. "Nice talking with you. *Toksha.*"

He walked to his daughter, then turned and smiled to Somay and me.

"I'm always struck by the feeling native peoples have for the Holocaust," I said. "The first time I came here, your father told me that he regarded the Reservations as 'concentration camps.' When I told my wife, she compared the Reservations to more like 'ghettos', and said that, unlike Hitler, the American government never could quite 'pulled the trigger' when it came to doing away with native peoples."

"The government might not have 'pushed that button' on exterminating all of us, but Hitler got many of his ideas from the United States," she responded. "He studied the Reservation system when he was making his plans. 'Blood quantum' and determining who was a Jew - Hitler didn't just make that up; he got all that from the way this government decided it for our people. Fifty percent – and you were an Indian; twenty-five percent – and you were white. Hitler used those same percentages for deciding which Jews would live and which would die. In California, the government actually paid people to kill the natives there. It was written into law."

I looked at her, aghast and disgusted. I would have never thought in my lovely State of California such inhumanity could have existed.

"They were conquerors," she said.

Murderers, I thought.

A shallow feeling gripped my chest.

How could I be so insensitive? How could I have spoken the way I did?

I realized that my view of the government came from an entirely different perspective than hers. Unlike the experience of her people, this country had saved mine. I held that if it hadn't been for the United States intervening in World War II, I wouldn't be here, and the Jewish people wiped out – erased from this earth.

This country had given me and my family life, land, that no doubt native peoples had been pushed off of. Their land.

My heart sank in my chest. I wanted to ask forgiveness, but stood quiet, not knowing what to do.

Certain I'd spoiled the evening, I asked if she wanted to leave?

"No," she responded. "I think I'd like to dance."

I followed her onto the dancefloor. Her movements were fluid and graceful; a thing of beauty and wonder to behold. They spoke of femininity, and seemed to emanate a certain security and comfort from within.

She didn't need me, I thought. No one was about to ask her to step off the dancefloor if she weren't with a partner. No one would look at her the least bit strange dancing unaccompanied.

And I didn't want to introduce anything to our relationship; I didn't want to feel like I needed to give her my attention.

She turned, and we danced together – thoughts entering my head. How do I honor this person? How do I honor this moment? How can I treat her in the least possessive way possible and still somehow acknowledge that I feel so happy – so blessed – that she's graced me this way?

There's every reason for divides between us, I continued thinking. The color of my skin, my age, the fact I'm married.

Exiting the dancefloor, the bridesmaid smiled.

"The two of you are really good dancers," she said. "It was really nice to watch. Especially when the two of you got together. It was like you were so in sync with each other…"

CHAPTER SEVENTY

At the hotel April and I entered the ballroom. There was still dancing, and April wanted to join the others on the dancefloor; but I found an excuse, and we sat at a table. When I rose, I found my feet were bare, and my pants were missing.

"Do you know how we can get parking for the hospital, Dr. Mike?"

It was Somay.

No, I don't, I responded.

She looked confused.

"Aren't you a doctor there?" she asked.

Yes, I'm a doctor, I responded, but I don't know anything about parking.

She looked at me, doubtful...

Walking beside Somay along the hotel corridor, the walls were glass, so to be able to see within the rooms. Each room was occupied by a different couple; for some, the curtains were closed, concealing those within; for others, the curtains were parted, the couples like actors on an open stage. There was every kind of couple: straight, gay, interracial. Near the end of the hallway, the two final couples each consisted of an older man and younger woman...

Awakening from the dream, I pondered its meaning?

I didn't think I felt that way about Somay, but maybe I was mistaken?...

CHAPTER SEVENTY-ONE

At the hospital I passed Dr. Curtiz in the hall.

"I heard you were at a party with Orville White Buffalo's daughter," he said, smiling. "Yeah, news about that kind of thing travels fast around these parts. The moccasin telegraph is alive and well."

He looked to the side, then edged closer.

"There's something about Somay that I think you ought to know about," he said. "She may not be what she seems... For years she was struggling with chronic pain... She had a really bad case of meningitis early in life; then, she had an accident, and had to have surgery on her neck. She was getting Methadone to control the pain. Then, one of the urine drug screens came back positive for Meth."

"The confirmatory tests never did come back positive," he continued. "Ultimately, she took herself off the Methadone – Said she didn't want to be on it – Didn't like the way it made her feel."

"Anyway, you might want to keep your distance where Somay is concerned," he concluded. "I'd hate to see you get hurt..."

CHAPTER SEVENTY-TWO

Over the past weeks I'd made a habit of going to Somay's after work and collecting she and Wesley for a walk with Ini.

"Wesley's with dad," Somay said. "I'll let him know you came by."

"Is your car back from the shop?" I asked.

"Yes," she said, pointing at where it was parked behind the house. "It's running fine now."

Ini lunged and jumped at Somay; Somay held her paws.

"Going to dance with me, Ini?" she said. "Gonna dance?"

Ini caught the neck of Somay shirt and exposed a coin-sized burn above the breast-line.

"I fell asleep in bed, smoking a cigarette," she said.

I hadn't known she smoked.

"Yeah, bad habit," she said. "I fall back on it sometimes."

The wound was shaped like a malformed half-moon, the flesh bright pink.

How do you sleep through that? I thought, suspiciously…

CHAPTER SEVENTY-THREE

With the advent of spring, the snow receded, and the buffalo grass grew high; native plants were blooming, so that sage populated the land, as well as bushes full of choke-cherries and long strings of Indian turnips hidden underground.

But all the beauties of the nature were divorced of me, as dark clouds circled in my head.

Dr. Curtiz is right, I thought. What have I been doing? Coming around Somay's? It was wrong. I'd made myself too familiar. I was asking for trouble.

A moment later, though, my thoughts shifted to Wesley.

What would I tell him? What will he think if I don't come around anymore?

And what about Ini? To her, Somay is mom.

My thoughts harkened back to the blizzard, when Somay came and found us in the white-out. I thought of Tom Eagle and how he'd been lost in storm. It's possible that we owed her our lives.

Be reasonable, I thought. Consider what she's been through. The meningitis. The neck surgery. I hadn't a clue what is was to be in her shoes. I had no basis to compare. And even if I would have done things differently, I was in no position to judge. I wasn't brought up the way she was – With limited options compared to the ones I knew...

Curtiz said the Meth in her urine had never been confirmed. The whole allegation was unsubstantiated.

Probably, a false positive, I concluded. He had no right to even mention it – Should have never told me.

131

And who knows? Maybe, Somay wouldn't even notice if Ini and I didn't come around anymore? Who was I to her? She knew I was married.

Walking between the trees, I realized I'd lost track of Ini. I looked from side to side, but didn't see her. Then, I turned and found her trailing some twenty steps behind. Head bent, ears low, she was walking with what seemed a slight limp.

Had she hurt herself? I thought.

Examining her I looked for the presence of a wound or thorn or burr in her paw, but found nothing.

Resuming our walk I noticed what appeared like a couple fast paced shadows between the trees. Then, a coyote appeared. It was small and dainty, and I was reminded of the comments about Ini looking like a coyote. Turning, Ini was still lagging behind me. I reached for my cell phone to take a picture; but just as I was about to snap a photo, the coyote casually trotted off.

Darn, I thought. Just missed it.

Then, looking back to Ini, she was no longer behind me and nowhere to be found.

That's funny, I thought. I didn't see her go after the coyote.

Deciding there was no time for deliberations, I ran in the direction the coyote was heading, shouting for Ini – But all I found was open field.

Desperate, I called Somay.

"Oh, I think I hear something," she responded. "Yes, Ini is here."

I hurried back to her home.

"I'm glad you called me," she said. "Or else I wouldn't have heard the barking... Bad barking. I don't know if I would've went to the door."

"When I opened the door, there was Ini – run, run, run – and these two guys on the other side of the road. They said two coyotes were hot on her trail. They said they saw you running in the wrong direction."

'They saw me'? I repeated, incredulously.

"Yes," she responded. "I wish I had gotten more information, but instead of going after them, I was inspecting Ini. They basically implied that the coyot's almost got her – That they were awfully close. 'They were right on her heels,' they said."

It didn't make sense, I thought. They saw me at the river? That was a relatively long distance from here. Why would they follow her? Why hadn't they called to me? Said, "Over here, over here. Your dog is over here"? If they saw the whole thing - Me going in the wrong direction - They must have heard me call out. I was calling out at the top of my lungs. Why wouldn't they call back and alert me that they'd seen Ini? And how did they get here so quick?

"If I saw a dog being chased by a coyote, Dr. Mike, I would follow," Somay commented. "I can't believe I didn't talk with them more. They must have been standing right here. But by the time I saw there weren't any clear bite marks on her, they were gone.

"I did feel wet spots on her neck. There was spit on her neck and flank. That's where they go. They bite your neck. They'll bite at your flank. They will bite at your Achilles.

"I think somebody got her, but didn't score on the skin. There's no blood, though it feels a little swollen. There's also something wet here by her leg, but I wasn't sure if that was from her running – because she ran for her life."

"Her fur is so thick, you can't see it," she continued. "I can't be sure she doesn't have a small puncture wound, but it looks like it wasn't enough to get her to bleed. Hopefully she was able to evade to keep the bites from being more successful. Hopefully, she was doing her evading technique, where she can change direction on a dime.

"And she was all shook up when she got here, so that's why I was like focusing on her and making sure there weren't any clear bite marks – because she was shaking.

"I'm glad you reached me. I was about to go to my studio. If I had, she would have been out there with the coyotes..."

Thinking about it, I shuddered.

"Those people?" she continued. "I wish I'd gotten their names."

Did you know them? I asked.

"No," she responded. "I've never seen them before. But when they told me what they saw, I got all focused on Ini, and I stopped asking them anything."

"Maybe you can catch up with those two people?" she asked. "They were walking down the road after they told me what happened. Maybe you want to talk with them and ask them what happened yourself?"

Looking up the road, I thought I saw a couple figures ahead and ran after them at full speed, calling out.

I lost sight of them just after they crossed a small footbridge, and, in their place, a coyote trotted out, and then another.

The two showed no sign of fear. Indeed, as I stood my ground, I had the feeling of being circled by sharks.

Looking back, I saw Somay; she had followed me and was holding Ini close to her side.

"There they are, Dr. Mike," she said. "The coyot's. They're right there. They're looking at us. They're so big."

Yes, these coyot's weren't like the one I tried to photograph; whereas that one looked dainty and delicate, these were like wolves.

"That's what they do," Somay commented. "They send in the smallest, youngest one to make the dog curious. Then, they go after the dog – Ambush the dog."

Still, I was surprised they'd go after Ini.

"Maybe they saw that the two of you were separated?" she responded. "They were probably hungry. They've been riding out the storms outside."

But Ini and I couldn't have been more than 20-feet apart.

"Yeah, but maybe the coyotes were angling her in a certain way, and they separated you," she said. "Ini probably knew that if she would've crossed that 20 feet to you, those coyotes would've intercepted her and brought her down and killed her right there. She probably made that decision in a split second. 'Too dangerous to go to dad. I've got to run.'"

I looked at Ini and recalled that she hadn't growled at the small coyote or run after it as she'd done with coyotes on other occasions.

"She probably knew that you were surrounded," Somay said. "You didn't know it, but she did. It was an ambush. They probably knew the two of you. Probably seen you guys walk those trails hundreds of times."

I shook my head. I couldn't believe I'd failed her that way.

"But you called me, Dr. Mike," Somay said. "And I opened the door, and she was there. Those people said the coyot's were still circling around her…"

In the evening I related the day's events to April.

"She's really smart," she said of Ini. "She ran to Somay's."

Why wouldn't she have just stayed with me? I asked. Instead of running off?

"She probably wanted to lead them away from you," she responded.

I nodded. Considering the size of those two larger coyotes, they probably would have torn me apart, too, had I interfered.

"So it's probably a good thing what happened," April added. "She veered them off basically is what she did.

I told her about the two men who'd supposedly witnessed the chase.

"Sounds like they were guardian angels," April commented.

"But it was odd," I replied, doubtful. "Because I went running after them, and thought I saw them, and then, in their place, came these two coyot's?..."

I related what Dr. Curtiz had told me earlier in the day and how conflicted I was.

"Whatever it is," April concluded, "you better get right with the spirits again..."

CHAPTER SEVENTY-FOUR

During the night Ini walked with a limp.

I re-examined her for wounds, but still found nothing there.

Probably from being chased by those coyotes, I thought.

As the hours passed, her limp became more pronounced and when I palpated for a strained muscle, she flinched, then took to her bed and stayed there. I could hear her stomach grumble, but she neither ate nor drank and in the morning she still hadn't touch her food or water.

"Com' on, Ini," I said. "Eat something."

Then, a knock came from the door. Opening it Orville stood on the porch.

"How you doing, Dr. Mike?" he said. "Just thought I'd see how you've been. I heard we missed you yesterday when you and Ini came around looking for Wesley. He says hello. Somay told me about the coyotes that chased Ini."

Ini limped towards him.

"How's my little coyot'?" he said, smiling.

I don't know that those coyotes felt all that 'akin' to her, I responded. More like they were intent on consuming her.

Orville laughed.

"In the old days, sometimes a female coyote would lore the dogs," he said. "When a coyote female would go into heat, it would attract the male dogs. There was interbreeding – here and all over."

Nodding, I told Orville that Ini was limping again, and hadn't ate or drank.

"Hmmm," he responded. "Something the matter, Doc?"

I looked at him, confused. What would there be something the matter with me for? And what would that have to do with Ini?

"The dog has a much closer relationship to the senses than we do," he continued. "It's because they live closer to Mother Earth, being that they move on four legs, while we move standing upright on two. We learn a lot from them, by just watching them. If there's anything or anyone who has compassion or forgiveness, it's the dog first. We, as two-leggeds... Well, we can get over that; but we harbor anger for long, long periods of time. So they teach us forgiveness – compassion – the ability to rely on each other. They have that, and they teach us those kinds of gifts. They sense how you're feeling. It's not by just looking at you. She knows your senses. She knows if you're happy. She knows if you're bewildered – if you're in deep thought – if you're pondering over something, and you can't find an answer – if you're frustrated. She's going to sense it. To keep her distance until you talk to her – and make her understand. I think if you do that, she'll understand. I hope she will."

"Those are the things that we are taught as young people in our childhood," he concluded. "'Learn to forgive.' A dog will forgive you every time. Except if you train it different – you train it to protect itself, so you build walls. Some of them are raised that way – And it's not right, but people do take advantage of their spirit. And they hurt that way. It's like committing a homicidal act, when they should be treated like companions – members of the family. We interrupt their lives with our own ignorance – and the outcome is either they become very sickly, or else they come out a very angry spirit..."

CHAPTER SEVENTY-FIVE

Outside, it was a beautiful spring day. Everything seemed to sparkle. The sky. The clouds. I looked at Ini. For the time being anyway, she wasn't limping. Opening the door, she followed me out. I thought of Orville. All that wisdom and good counsel. And here I am intent on walling off his daughter.

Then, the memory of the conversation with Dr. Curtiz resurfaced.

I can't, I thought. I can't have anything to do with her.

Turning, Ini was trailing behind me again. Three deer appeared in front of us. The animals stood watching, flipping and signaling each other with their white tails. They didn't start to run until we were within some thirty feet of them. I looked back at Ini.

She must have seen them, I thought. They were running through the field in plain view!

Still, she didn't chase them and continued to trail behind.

Not far ahead we came upon a mound of prairie dogs. They were actively scurrying about. But Ini walked right past. Several of them stopped and looked inquisitively at Ini, as though wondering what was wrong?

My frustration is getting to her, I determined. She's the one paying the price. It's now been two days that she hasn't eaten. And more than walks or nature or sunrises or the promise of food or treats, it was me and my emotional state that would make the difference between pulling her out of this condition or not.

I turned and invited her to play. She looked at me, then sprang and tugged at my heel – and we played in the snow on this beautiful winters day.

Then, the thought of Dr. Curtiz's warning, and the dark mood settled over me again.

I'll have no further dealings with her, I thought. I will not interact with her again. I can't.

And looking behind Ini was trailing me again – ears lowered, body hunkered, expression pained.

"She's going to sense it. To keep her distance until you talk to her – and make her understand."

I have to let go of this mood. I have to let go of it for the sake of Ini.

And I need to do it for myself. This is no way to be. Suspecting another with no real basis. It's wrong!

I encouraged Ini to play again, and, in my head, gave voice to her thoughts.

You don't need to worry, Mike. Somay is good. Everything will be fine. You'll see.

It's you I worry about. That's why I'm not feeling good. That's why I'm not eating. It's because I'm worried about you. I'm worried.

I love you, Mike. I love you. Can't you see how much I love you? Can't you see?...

"Oh, I'm so glad you were able to get yourself out of that mood," April said. "I'm so glad you're taking care of yourself, so you can take care of her. She has that instinct in her that knows what's unhealthy. It can become very serious if dogs don't drink. There are some dogs that really can't survive without drinking for a few days."

"I'm sorry that Dr. Curtiz upset you," she continued. "You don't know what Somay's been through. It's not right to judge her. It's just not..."

CHAPTER SEVENTY-SIX

In the morning I awoke to the staccato sound of thumping on the hardwood floor. I recognized it as Ini limping. In the kitchen Ini looked up at me, vulnerable.

"Ini, let me work on your muscles," I said.

But the moment I so much as touched the muscles around her leg, she flinched and pulled away.

Frustrated, I looked at her disapprovingly.

"Ini, you can't go on this way," I said. "Look at you with your gimpy little leg. You have to stand strong. Not like that – with it turned out like a ballet dancer. I'm getting past my injury – you have to get past yours!"

After a few more attempts, I didn't have the heart to try again. I reached for the phone and called Somay.

"She won't stop limping," I said. "It's as bad as it ever was before, and seems to have to do something with her iliopsoas muscle... It's a really deep muscle that stretches from the back all the way to the hip. I don't know how it got activated. Every time I so much as touch around there, Ini jumps and pulls away. Will you help me do some ischemic compression with her?..."

At Somay's we worked on Ini together. Knots in the muscles released and, afterwards, Ini's walked more normal.

How deep does it go? I thought. How long will she require treatment? I would have expected the muscles to be better by now. But, still, the issues with her leg continue. It feels like it's taking her so long to heal and it's still ongoing. The injury occurred when she was probably less than six months old and here we are six months later. In dog years, it translates to the injury occurring when she was three, and at age seven she's still healing from it.

I shook my head.
It's like healing is a lifelong matter...

CHAPTER SEVENTY-SEVEN

Leaving the house, the four of us – Somay, Wesley, Ini and me – took a walk along the river. Coming around a bend, Wesley spotted a mound of prairie dogs.

"Com'on, Ini!" Wesley said. "Let's get'em!"

He ran toward the mound; Ini not far behind.

"Raaahhh!" Wesley roared, as he and Ini swooped in.

But the lithe, little creatures just dove into the mound, well ahead of their pursuers. Smiling, I turned to Somay.

"Funny, the things little boys think," I said.

The words jogged the memory of my last camping trip with Chrissie.

"She was my uncle's girlfriend," I said. "We were sitting at the campfire – Chrissie, my uncle, brother and me. I couldn't have been much older than Wesley at the time. Other camping trips my uncle would bring his short-wave radio, and we'd listen to ghost stories. He didn't this time, so I decided to try to tell one. When I finished, Chrissie leans back and says, 'Ugh, why do children tell such stupid stories?'"

I shook my head.

"That was the next to last night I saw her alive."

"What happened to her?" Somay asked.

I shrugged.

"She killed herself," I responded. "I found out when I overheard my uncle talking on the phone one day. He was saying something about Chrissie's dog, Brie. 'What do you need to find a home for Brie for?' I asked. 'Because Chrissie died,' he said. 'She took a lot of pain pills and killed herself.' I blamed myself for years."

"Why?" Somay said. "Had you been bad to her?"

No, nothing like that, I responded. It was because I felt like we'd contributed to their breakup.

"When my parents divorced," I explained, "my uncle took us under his wing, becoming something of a father figure to my brother and me. I don't think Chrissie was too excited about it. The first time he took us to their apartment, she emerged from a beaded hallway completely naked."

"Why did she do that?" Somay asked.

"I don't know," I said. "Maybe it was her way of saying, 'This is my place, and – young children or not – I'm not going to change.'"

"Was she mean to you?" she asked.

"I wouldn't say 'mean'," I responded. "Just distant."

My thoughts drifted back to that last camping trip. The tent near a stream; sunlight twinkling off the water; the fresh taste of cool, mountain spring water in my mouth. Then, sitting around the campfire; Chrissie opposite me; wearing green shorts and hiking boots; her body illuminated by the fire; leaning against a log; glaring at me.

"Why do you think people have children?" she demanded.

I shrugged.

"Maybe because they want company?" I responded, uncertain.

She threw her head back, her eyes closed to all the stars in the heavens above in the night sky.

"That's selfish!" she asserted. "If you want company, get a dog!"

I looked at Somay. She was wearing shorts and hiking boots – the same as Chrissie. I recalled she'd been wearing them the first day we met. Perhaps that's why I experienced that immediate feeling of familiarity for her?

"The following day," I continued, "we went for a long hike in the woods. Coming back to camp, I remembered smiling – feeling really happy. My uncle had promised that we'd go fishing when we got back to camp. I'd been looking forward to that the whole trip. I could hardly contain my excitement."

As we ambled on, a thin chain tethered between two trees came into view. At its lowest point, the chain was hanging perhaps a foot from the ground, and seeing it, my brother ran ahead.

"Watch me," he called out. "I'm going to jump over it."

"Joe, you come back here!" my uncle shouted.

"Oh, let him be," Chrissie said, annoyed.

Joe ran and leapt, but caught his toe after almost clearing the chain. He tumbled in a heap, but got up again, unscathed; he dusted himself off, and continued his merry way as though nothing happened.

"You see," Chrissie said, triumphant. "He fell. He's okay."

But my uncle's featured darkened. It was a look I knew well, and felt afraid for Chrissie, because I knew harsh words usually followed.

"Listen," he said, "when you have children, you can let them run and jump and hurt themselves all you want. But I'm in charge of these kids, and they'll do what I say."

"But as long as you've 'fixed' yourself," he added, "you have nothing to say about it."

Arriving back at camp, I immediately set about assembling my fishing pole. Then, my uncle appeared, trudging through the campgrounds, announcing we were breaking camp.

"Why, Uncle Gary?" I asked.

"Because Chrissie wants to go home," he responded.

The drive felt like an eternity. Chrissie's dog, Brie, a German shepherd, drooling on me as the cool breeze poured in through the open window.

Finally, we stopped at what looked like a large log cabin. Inside, there was a bar; men pleasantly conversing over a drink. A hostess led us between tables until seating us near a wooden stage. Chrissie's features softened as she looked out.

"I used to dance at a place like this," she said. "I fell off a stage not very different from this one and hurt my leg."

As I looked at the stage, the image of her falling left me feeling sad.

"Is the reason you wanted to leave early because of what Uncle Gary told you?" I asked.

"That's part of it," she said, matter-of-factly.

I turned. Looking out my eyes settling on a plain-looking woman at another table, who sat pleasantly listening to conversation, before breaking into friendly laughter.

I turned back to Chrissie.

"What will happen now?" I asked.

"I don't know," she responded. "This might be our last supper..."

"When my uncle told me about Chrissie's death," I said, "my mind flashed to that walk to the campsite – their argument – and what she told me at the restaurant. I turned to him, looking for reassurance. 'Was the reason the two of you broke up because of Joe and me?' I asked. 'That was part of it,' he responded."

"Did your uncle ever marry?" Somay asked.

"Yeah," I replied, absently. "Yeah, he did. My Aunt Glenda. As a matter of fact – years later – he told me he'd just begun dating

Glenda when Chrissie called, and sounded so ill he told Glenda he had to go to her.

"When he got there, he said she looked terrible; hadn't taken care of herself; hadn't taken care of the dog; the place was a mess. So, he cleaned the apartment; cooked for her; talked; said he wasn't a therapist, but tried to do the things a friend would do.

"He said Chrissie was a 'sad' person. That she'd been in counselling for years, but could never quite put her demons behind her.

"He was checking on her every day after that. Then, when he came around the sixth day, he said she looked a lot better – like her usual self again. The place was clean, table set, she'd even cooked a meal. 'Well, this is a change,' he says.

"Afterwards, she tells him some guy has invited her over for the weekend, and asks what he thought she should do? 'Yeah, sure,' he says. 'Sounds like a good idea. You could get out.'

"Not long after, he gets a call from the apartment manager, saying the dog was inside barking, and wouldn't stop. When he got there, they opened the door together, and found her laying on the bed. She'd taken narcotics for years following that dance hall injury. There were empty bottles all around her."

I hesitated.

"He said he'd nearly come the day before," I continued. "Been planning to show her his new car.

"But, on the way, he got a call – Told her he had to do something – And have to take a 'raincheck.'

"Afterward, he kept asking himself, 'What if I'd gone over that day? Would it have made a difference? Could I have stopped her?'

"He said for a long time after that, any time he saw a red-head with Chrissie's general physique and complexion, he'd have to look into her face to convince himself it wasn't her. He could be driving on the highway, and if a woman with red hair passed him, he'd follow her. It could take him miles out of his way. It didn't matter. He wouldn't stop. Not until he caught up with her, looked at her face, and could be sure it wasn't Chrissie.

"'I buried that woman,' he told me. 'I put her in the ground, and covered her up. And, still, every time I saw a woman that looked like Chrissie, I had to follow her until I could be sure it wasn't her.' I don't even know how long that lasted? Maybe years?"

I broke off.

"When we talked, he said he recalled a morning when the two of them were sitting at the kitchen table. Chrissie says, 'Why don't we get married?' This woman who he loved.

"He shook his head, though. 'I don't think that's such a good idea,' he responded. Too much baggage, he told me."

I looked out at the natural beauty all around us.

"I wish he would have married her. I wish he would have seized the moment those last days they were together and proposed. Because he loved her. And she loved him."

"Like you and your wife," Somay responded.

I gasped, a misplaced smile gracing my features.

"More than you know," I said...

CHAPTER SEVENTY-EIGHT

At the Juvenile Detention Center I accompanied Orville. He taught a class there in the afternoons, and I was interested in attending. Surrounded by a high barbed wire fence, there were bars on all the windows, and emanated an eerie silence. Making our way through the entrance, Orville leaned heavily on the front counter, peered through the window at the guard, and spoke through a slit in the bullet proof glass.

"I'm here for the class," he said, breathless.

The guard said nothing; buzzing us in through the heavy steel and glass door, he escorted us through the hallway to the classroom. The space felt tight and confined; every noise seemed vibrated through all quarters, as though even sound could not escape there. I sat in the back, and watched as the young inmates filed in. They lumbered between the aisles till slouching into an available chair. Orville sat in the front, waiting patiently; his expression revealing no hint of judgment or concern for time.

"I wanted to tell you guys a story," he began. "About my friend Jimmy. He was a Blackfoot Indian. He was a movie actor. I met him in L.A. I was twenty. I was working as a drywall hanger. We'd get together on weekends and visit. We'd go together to the Indian bars. There were a lot of Indian bars in LA in those days. Sometimes, you go in one and it was just like you're on the reservation. One time, we went into this huge bar, and I was walking through, and somebody calls, 'Hey, Tihansi.' That means 'cousin.' I turned around and it's an Indian guy, and he's not even Lakota, but he knew what word to use to get your attention.

"Well, one day Jimmy gives me an invitation for a party in Hollywood. So, that weekend, after I got paid, I asked a taxi to take me to that address. It took me to a residential area. Beautiful homes. There was a table as long as this room – any drink you wanted. Then, another table – just as long – with any drug you wanted.

"So I grabbed a can of Budweiser, and I was visiting around. Then, I went over and I was looking at the drugs – so many different colored pills, hash, and all kinds of stuff. Then, Jimmy came over. He called me 'Kola' – it means 'friend.' He said, 'Kola, did you ever try those?' 'No,' I said, 'I don't even know what that they are. I've heard of them, but I've never tried it.' He said, 'Someone here is going to offer you something. But you and I were born and raised on an Indian Reservation. There's a lot of things we lock up in here.' He pointed to his heart. 'Inside of us. A lot of anger, frustrations in there,' he said. 'We get into that, down the road, we'll either kill somebody, or we'll kill ourselves. Because what's inside is going to come out.' He lifted his hand like a plume of rising smoke. 'And we got to handle that,' he said, emphatically, *'the right way'...*"

CHAPTER SEVENTY-NINE

"I remember when I was your guys' age," Orville continued. "It was in the 1960s, after I came out of high school. I graduated in 1959. There was no talk about college. I came out of a boarding school with a third grade level of education and total dependency on authority. You know what that means? It means you can't function without consent. You feel like you always have to go to someone before you make a decision. You need someone else to say, 'This is what you should do.'

"When I was in my senior year, a BIA worker came. He said, 'What you want to do after you graduate?' I said, 'What you mean?' He said, 'You can go to school.' I said, 'What kind of school?' He said, 'Well, you can be a carpenter, auto mechanic, painter, plumber.' I said, 'I want to be an x-ray lab technician.' And, boy, he just sat back and said, 'But you people are so good with your hands.' I heard that so many times since then – nothing about the mind – 'You people are so good with your hands.'

"Well, I said, 'I'd like to try this.' He said, 'Let's look at your transcript.' So he got the copies of my high school transcript. I went in that boarding school when I was in eighth grade. I barely spoke English. They put me in with the eighth-graders because of my age. And I just passed along.

"In my transcript it showed that I was an average to above average student. Junior and senior year I made the honor role at least twice. He looked at it and said, 'Well, maybe, you can handle it.'

"He said, 'You have three choices. You can go to Dallas, Chicago, or Los Angeles.' He might as well said, 'You can go to the moon' - because the furthest I'd been from the Reservation was Nebraska for the harvest, and I'd never been in the city.

"I thought about it, and I picked Dallas, Texas. In July 1959, I walked into the Parkland Memorial Hospital, and found out that I barely spoke English, I had very simple understanding of math, I didn't even know what science courses were. Not biology, nothing. I never felt so stupid in my life.

"I did the manual things, like developing films, mixing solutions. But when it came to reading, I didn't know what I was reading. Because I wasn't that fluent in English.

"So I quit. Afterwards, I worked there for over a month till I made enough to buy a ticket for a bus and came back to the Reservation.

"And that idea of having a wonderful transcript when you don't know nothing – boy, that really hurt. I came home thinking that I was just dumb..."

CHAPTER EIGHTY

"I ended up back on the ranch," Orville continued. "Throughout high school I worked every summer for the ranchers south of Valentine. One of my brothers and I would break and train horses for the ranchers. So I went back to that. And I wondered if that was going to be my life. Because there really was no future in it.

"I spent a lot of time blaming God. In the boarding school the missionaries teach you that God has the answer to everything. So I blamed God for my failures. Until I said, 'Hey, it's my life. I gotta take charge.'

"And the thing that saved me was the stories that I grew up with in Spring Creek. In wintertime my mother and the elders of the community would tell stories. These were the ones who influenced me. Evenings were for storytelling. So we used to select our storyteller; we go over there during the day, and chop wood for them for the night; bring water for them. Then, we'd go home and eat, and later we'd come back; and one of us would roll some tobacco, light it, and offer it to the storyteller. Then, for about an hour – an hour and a half – they would tell stories. That's where we learned where we came from; about medicine men and women. That's where we learned about spirits, and what spirits are and how to work with them.

"And they talked about our grandfathers on a *Zuya*. That means 'life's journey' – the experiences they had in that journey, and how they survived, and what they learned. In those days when a young boy reaches puberty, he is a man. He's not a boy anymore. There's no concept of teenage. He is a man. And part of being a man is making *Zuya*. Sometimes, they would be gone for months, years – depending on how far they go, or how long they stay out. But when they come home, they're fully mature, they saw what's out there in the world, they learned.

"So I heard those stories until I was sixteen, and was sent to the boarding school system. That was the same year that my mother died. My father had died when I was four, so, after that, I really didn't have any parents.

"In 1880 United States Congress passed a law outlawing all Indian spiritual practices. And they really enforced that. They take you into the boarding school usually when you're five years old, and they teach you to forget your language and anything you were brought up with.

"But I remembered the *Zuya* stories. So I went on my own *Zuya…*"

CHAPTER EIGHTY-ONE

"That's how I wound up in LA," he continued, "where I met Jimmy. I wondered what he meant by 'the right way.' Then, when I came back here, I met a medicine man, and he invited me to a sweat lodge ceremony. I had never known a medicine man. I never seen one when I was growing up – my aunts and uncles would have a sweat, but then they'd take the lodge apart. I was a little guy, just watching from a distance, and wouldn't pay no attention.

"So, I asked him why he wanted me to come to the ceremony? He said it was because he wanted me to translate for him – for those who can't speak Lakota. I asked him, 'Why do you want me to do that?' 'So, the people won't be afraid,' he said. 'So the people will not be afraid of us. People are afraid were talking with ghosts. But were not working with those things. We're working with relatives. If they know us, and what we have, and understand our altar, they will not be afraid.'

"I remember my first time in the sweat lodge. I went in that sweat lodge and I was sitting in there just like an Indian – cross-legged, with my arms crossed. And when they poured that water over the hot stones, that steam hit me right in the face – like a water balloon busts in your face. And I sucked in that hot air, and it blocked my windpipe, nose and throat. I almost panicked. I had to really concentrate, so I didn't run out of there.

"I went through the ceremony; when I came out, the inside of my mouth and nose were blistered, 'cause I inhaled that hot steam. The next day, though, I went back. This time, when I was inside with them, I really watched the others. As soon as they closed the door, I saw that all the guys went down. So, that's what I did – and bent my head down. The steam went over my head, and I didn't breathe it in.

153

And I went back again and again. Every time I went back, I learned a little more, because they explained a little more. Because just knowledge doesn't work, you have to experience these ways before you can understand it. And it really helped me. Somehow, it pulled me back. These medicine men helped pulled me back to my ways.

"These medicine men were all practicing underground. Nobody knew they were practicing. They had their own followers, families. And then they began teaching me. And as I sat in those ceremonies, I began thinking, 'That's what Jimmy was talking about.' He said, 'There are ways to find yourself. And if you do it right, it comes...'"

CHAPTER EIGHTY-TWO

"That law they passed outlawing all Indian spiritual practices," Orville said. "They really enforced that. When I went through that school system, it was evil to be an Indian. They would tell me, 'You speak of backwards language. You're savages. You need to be civilized.' That's all I learned in school – how bad I was.

"Most had been in that institution since they were five years old. So, by the time they were teenagers, they had already been conditioned to deny their Indian-ness. It really worked, too. On Saturdays, the school had Western movies. John Wayne. It was really funny, because we used to sit there and cheer for the Cowboys and the cavalry when they fought Indians. And we laughed at the Indians. That's how well the boarding school experience worked. Because you're in there since you were five years old, and that's the way they raise you.

"I was sixteen when they put me into a boarding school. I couldn't believe what was going on. I saw physical punishment, verbal punishment. This was in the 1950s. They developed punishments to get the message across. They really whipped you into submission. For some, you can still see the scars – where ears were ripped from the skin. That's why the older people here don't pass the language on to the children. Because they're afraid for them. Because they don't want them to be hurt in school.

"But I remember growing up in Spring Creek, where we were very free. We spoke our language day in and day out. We played in our language. We sang. We danced. We were happy. We laughed in our language.

"I talked to other elders who are fluent Lakota speakers, and I mentioned teaching our language to the children. They told me, 'Forget it. When we die, that's it.'

"And that's when I panicked. I thought, 'We can't lose this.' That's why I taught it to my children. That's why I'm teaching it to my grandson. That's why I'm here teaching it to you."

"I want you to know that I believe in you fellas," he concluded. "I believe you have it in you to be our next leaders. And we need leaders, because the people are hurting."

He stood, slowly.

"Okay, that's it for the day," he said. "See you tomorrow. *Toksha.*"

The young men filed out as they come in – heads down and silent. After the last of them had left, I approached Orville.

"That was really moving," I said. "Do you always talk with them this way?"

"Yeah," he said. "That's what I usually do."

That's amazing, I thought. In the span of less than an hour it felt like I had traveled and bore witness to a life's journey.

Arriving home, Ryan was out front working on his truck.

"I hear you're going with Orville to his classes," he said. "I'm glad. I think one of the big problems for our young people on the Reservation is feeling disconnected. When you disconnect people from their culture, their traditions, their ancestors, their families, that's when they'll give up. They use that as a tool for oppression. They know why they're disconnecting our young people and removing their culture... Because they understand that it makes them easier to control and able to be manipulated and, in the end, not want to be here anymore..."

CHAPTER EIGHTY-THREE

At the Standing Elk Park I went wading in the river. The river was as pristine as I remembered, and there was that same air of mystery. Not long after beginning to wade, I came upon a sandbar and found some enormous bird foot-prints there.

Someone breeding ostriches? I thought.

Ini mostly stayed on the shore watching me with concern; entering the water every so often and silently swimming after me, as though meaning for me to follow. At one point I looked back and didn't see her on the shore.

Where is she? I thought. Then, I felt a nudge to the side furthest from shore – and found Ini swimming around me, as though attempting to lasso me back.

In a bend of the river the water suddenly became deep. The badlands silt that usually coated the river floor had no way of anchoring itself against the swift current, leaving only smooth bedrock underneath. Ini and I had nothing to grip and went sliding on the river floor. Caught up in the current, we were swept down the river, till deposited on the other side of the bank.

I probed the river for a shallow place to cross back again. Ini had been watching me from shore; then, she embarked on entering the water and swimming ahead of me – as she typically preferred to be the one to scout ahead.

But in this circumstance, the current was too much for her, and she was swept down the river, until finally climbing back ashore.

Ini shook herself off, then sent a chorus of barks in my direction.

"I can't get across," she seemed to say. "The current is too strong for me."

Indeed, I could find no shallow place; everywhere the water level was up to my navel.

Still, as it seemed there was nothing to do but ford the river, I made my way back to Ini. At first she appeared happy to see me. Then, recognizing my intent, she took several steps back. But there was nothing to do but collect her and attempt to cross. Ini noticeably trembled.

This dog that walks out into blizzards without a moment's hesitation, I thought. And now she's shaking.

I steadied myself with each step, in silent prayer that I would keep my companion safe.

Then, in front of us, appeared the largest blue heron I'd ever seen.

The giant bird tracks! I thought. I'd found the source!

Smiling, I walked towards the bird. It watched us; and although offering no expression recognizable by me, it didn't leave until we were safely across. Then, with a wing-span stretching some six or seven feet, it took to the air and flew off into the horizon.

From the other side of the river, I looked back. There was the blinding light through the trees into the wide expanse of pristine, unspoiled natural beauty abound on the Reservation. A part of me didn't want to leave; but surrender to the flowing river forever....

CHAPTER EIGHTY-FOUR

At the clinic an inmate from the jail (dressed in an orange jumpsuit) was seated in the waiting area just outside my office. A guard escorted him into the examination room.

"Do you want me to stay?" the guard asked.

No, that's not necessary, I said.

The man was cuffed at the wrists and ankles.

"You can take those off, too," I said.

The guard proceeded to remove the shackles, then left the room. I leaned back in my chair and tried to be casual.

"What brings you here today?" I asked.

He shrugged.

"Nothing," he said. "I'm being transferred to Recovery. I just need medical clearance."

He talked about his struggles with drugs and alcohol.

"I feel like I was a set up for drug addiction," he said, "because of the home I grew up in. When I was coming up, my grandfather tried to help. He was a recovered addict himself. But he came from a long line of medicine men. He offered me a lot of wisdom. Things he knew and learned. He knew the old ways - taught me about the Lakota virtues. I think he did it because he knew what was ahead for me - because of what I was being exposed to. So, one day, I could get over addiction – heal myself. I think he was trying to save me."

My mind drifted as I thought of Wesley.

"He's dead now," he continued. "My grandpa. I think Mr. White Buffalo comes to the jail and teaches us for the same reason my grandpa taught me.

I nodded.

Yes, I agree, I said.

"You were at Mr. White Buffalo's Sweat," he said. "What did you think of the ceremony?"

I said they were helping me. When I was young, I nearly drowned; so anything that rekindles that feeling of not being able to breathe is difficult for me. But I found the ceremonies healing, and kept trying, till now I attend without difficulty.

"I think it's a good thing that you come," he said. "Makes guys inside feel like there's someone from the clinic who cares about our values."

He leaned back.

"Are you a Christian, Dr. Mike?" he asked.

No, I'm Jewish, I said. Though these days my wife was referring to me as a 'practicing Lakota.' He grinned.

"Have you been to Mr. White Buffalo's Sundance?" he asked. "Did you experience anything there?"

As a matter of fact, I had. It happened during the 'children's round.' As I stepped into the circle and approached the tree of life, I experienced this sensation of 'tearing' across the muscles of my chest – like there was some physical wound there for no reason. And when the round was over, the ache dissipated, and, in its place, was this feeling of deep relaxation and healing that spread over my chest.

"Spirit helpers," he responded. "That's what my grandfather would say. You were touched by a helper, because you were open to the experience. And the helper let you in, so you could understand it, and appreciate what was happening."

"When did you know you were going to come here, Dr. Mike?" he asked.

I shook my head, struggling for something to say other than events pertaining to my FQHC experience.

"I guess I had a dream about it," I said. "A native man standing in a doorway; calling out for water; running to him; but when I got there, his very substance had transformed and merged with the door; and reaching him, I, too, transformed, merging into the doorway."

Finishing my story, he was silent. I lowered my gaze.

How could I be so inappropriate? I thought. Here this patient comes to me for medical evaluation, and I'm telling him about dreams.

The guard came back in the room and re-applied the shackles. The patient shuffled out; but at the doorway, he turned.

"To our people," he said, "water is sacred. Running to a man calling out for water is to give nourishment. So, you came in service and melded into the doorway. And in that emersion, you became part of the threshold, too.

"I see you doing your part to fulfill your dream. Being of service. Bringing water to those who are parched. The challenge you face is that people don't usually stay in a doorway – you go through a doorway, and move on. You just have to understand your medicine. Because when you understand the medicine that you have, it makes it easier to live your life. Because you don't feel so torn, and pulled apart. And I'm not just talking about what they taught you in medical school – I'm talking about your intrinsic medicine."

Then, he turned, the guard leading him away...

CHAPTER EIGHTY-FIVE

With a stick he'd picked up along the way , Wesley played fetch with Ini. Then, on a stretch of trail where sticks were plentiful, Wesley picked up and threw so many that Ini had a hard time keeping up; as soon as Ini retrieved one, she was off chasing another. I thought she would get frustrated; but Ini just kept good-naturedly going back and forth.

"I think she likes Wesley's little boy energy," Somay said. "It's too bad your wife and you don't have kids."

Then, she stopped and suddenly got quiet.

"It's alright," I said.

I thought about the conversation with the inmate, and the things I didn't tell him.

"Coming here, I didn't have much choice," I said. "You might say I had to come back. It was about the only avenue I had left.

"I ran afoul with the clinic where I was working – a place called FQHC. I accepted the job there because April's grandmother was dying, and the clinic was nearby. The grandmother was all but mother to April; this way she could be there for her grandmother's final days.

"I was an experienced physician. Before FQHC I'd been a medical director with the Tennessee Health Department; I'd received commendations from Health Department for transforming the worst community medical center in the state to a model of excellence. Given those past achievements, I couldn't imagine having a problem at FQHC.

"But I guess you could say I didn't understand the ground rules. FQHC stands for Federally Qualified Health Center. They receive most of their funding from the government. I thought at a place like this, standard of care would be the norm. But the doctors there were doing a lot of questionable things. Tons of money wasted on unnecessary tests, referrals, and imaging studies. Worst of all was all the narcotic prescribing. Vicodin, Darvon, Percocet being doled out like candy. When I'd be asked to cover for these other doctors, I'd perform urine drug screens to determine if their patients were taking these medications appropriately. Inevitably, results showed that the narcotics weren't in their system – What was showing up was heroin and cocaine. And here FQHC was right next to a school. Instead of part of the solution, it felt like FQHC was part of the problem, and rather than working to keep national healthcare afloat, it was sinking it."

I shook my head.

"I was having nightmares," I continued. "In one of them, I was at a waterpark with my colleagues; they were sliding their children down waterslides. But instead of water, the slides were streaming blood, and all of them were covered in it. Looking at them, they were smiling; seemingly having a good time with their wives and children. I stood pleading, 'Guys, this isn't right.'"

"Do you typically act on your dreams, Dr. Mike?" Somay asked.

"Yes," I said. "I awoke from that dream knowing I had to do something... I went right to my Clinical Director and insisted he act to correct those problems."

She nodded.

"That's the reason why we dream," she said. "To work things out..."

CHAPTER EIGHTY-SIX

"Not long after I went to the Clinical Director," I continued, "I became the target for every kind of inquiry and investigation. They told me all my cases were being reviewed, and if a hundred percent didn't meet their satisfaction, I'd be terminated. Over the ensuing weeks, they really made an example out of me. They moved me from cubicle to cubicle. Put me in rooms right next to construction; sledgehammers operating essentially right next to me. Finally, they placed me on a forced leave of absence while they 'considered' my position. A week later I received my termination notice."

"How could they do that?" she asked. "When you were doing your job?"

"They could do what they wanted," I responded, matter-of-factly. "Even though it was a federally-qualified health center subsidized by the government, it was privately owned. I'd signed an 'at-will' contract in a 'right-to-work' state. I had no recourse."

"It's like the allegory of the cave," Somay said. "Do you remember that story?... There are these three men chained to the wall of a cave. They were born that way. And the only thing they ever knew was a fire that was up behind them. But they didn't know it was a fire– It was just something that would cast shadows on the wall. And so, their reality was the destruction of these shadows on the wall. And come one morning – well, they didn't really know what morning or night was, they only knew the shadows on the wall and the conversations they had between them – one day, one of the three looked down and found the shackles on his wrists had been removed. He goes, 'Wow, I can stand up.' So, he stood up. And the other two were still discussing the shadows on the wall. So, he turns around and see's that there's a fire on a ledge. And then, he looks over and sees that there's an opening to the cave, and walks out and sees the sun.

"The sun is the representation of enlightenment. And so he comes and he tells his friends – he says, 'This isn't the way it is. Your perception is singular. The only thing you know who is shadows, and there's a fire here, and if you go outside, there's a sun, and there's life, and there's enjoyment.'

"And what do they do? They kill him. They killed him because they were so afraid of the world, and how big it was, and there were things beyond the shadows of the cave.

"And that's the burden to society of enlightenment. And the burden of ignorance. So when you tell these stories, and you share these experiences, I think, 'So, Dr. Mike, was sharing these experiences with people who were only seeing shadows on the wall - people who weren't ready for enlightenment.'

"I think that's the problem you had at your previous place of work: It was that you see the sun, and these other people see the shadows. And it's because the world is sometimes too big for people, and it makes them feel uncomfortable, which is why capitalism is such a frenzy. If I go to a foreign place, it's easier to go to someplace I know, like McDonald's, then to eat the native food. It's different, so it's weird for people, and makes them uncomfortable, and feel queer, and awkward, and unsettled. So you could be bringing this enlightenment to your peers, and your peers are like, 'Why would you feel that way? I saw shadows. You say you saw something else.'

"In reality, you saw pain, and addiction, and these bad things that were happening to other people. And the fact that you can see that, you can empathize, and understand it from another's perspective.

"But people put you down for that, and said, 'Oh, there's nothing to that.' And that's too bad. Because by doing that, your peers were cashing in on others' pain…"

CHAPTER EIGHTY-SEVEN

"After being fired," I continued, "I couldn't find a clinic that would take me. My applications were near universally rejected. When I did get an interview and tried to explain what happened at FQHC, it was mostly received with skepticism. One interviewer told me, 'We typically don't do urine drug screens here – Bad for business.'

"I was still bound by my obligation to the National Health Service Corps. April and I spent our days on the phone with NHSC officials. In the end it didn't matter to them that I'd signed up as a matter of idealism – wanting to serve my country like the World War II veterans I'd cared for in Tennessee – with only $2000 worth of loans that they'd repaid. Between interest and time left on my commitment, the NHSC insisted I owed them hundreds of thousands. And, to them, it didn't matter the reason I was fired – Termination was a criteria for default. Placed in default with the government, I wouldn't be able to charge the Centers of Medicare & Medicaid for patient services. If that happened, I'd be un-hirable as a physician, and essentially unable to practice medicine.

"April tried to be supportive, but there were times her faith really faltered. 'All these doctors handing out narcotics and doing all these bad things to patients,' she said, 'but they still have jobs! And they're not sitting around, losing their jobs, calling lawyers, and not knowing how they're going to support their families.'

"We'd been trying to have children, but with everything happening, April felt like we had to put our plans on hold. Then, she was diagnosed with cancer."

In the meadow, daisies and other flowers were pushing up from the ground. Somay stopped by a bush with dark red berries.

"Chokecherries," she said. "Would you mind if I picked some? I used them for jams."

I thought I'd seen the same bush some weeks ago, but there weren't berries then?

"Yes, they only bloom a short time, and we're near the end of the season," she said.

Only fruitful for a season, I thought. And then the time is past.

"By choosing life for your patients – who didn't even want what you were offering them – you chose death for us."

I lowered my head. Somay stopped picking chokecherries, and crouched by the river...

CHAPTER EIGHTY-EIGHT

Holding his knee, the patient in the examination room sat in obvious discomfort.

"My knee is always swollen," he said. "Last time I came here, they had to drain it… I re-injured it a couple of months ago. It happened while I was helping my uncle fix a leak in his roof. I slipped off the ladder. For a while, I was just hanging there. I was lucky I didn't fall. "

I examined his knee; fluid filled, applying pressure on one side led to bulging on the other.

"Your knee needs elevation, anti-inflammatories, and rest until we can get you to the Orthopedists."

"You're not getting me to the Orthopedists," he responded. "I already got the letter from Contract Health saying there isn't any money."

He said the anti-inflammatories weren't work.

"All they're doing is upsetting my stomach," he said. "I had a bleeding ulcer back when I was drinking. That's when I quit. Alcoholism ruined my life. I've been sober for the past six months. Whenever I have the urge to drink, I go and be with people. Spending time in people's homes has been keeping me from going back to alcohol.

"I need to keep walking, doc. When I stop, the urge to drink comes back. So I go between homes of friends and family night, so I won't think about it, and I can fight that urged by talking.

"I used to walk seven miles a day. I go everywhere on my own two feet. It's the way I get my exercise. It's the way I got around to people on the Rez. Now, I can hardly walk at all.

"I love to cook for people. I cook at the school cafeteria. People invite me over to their homes to cook after ceremonies. Now, I can't get anywhere unless someone comes and picks me up."

"The Vicodin helped," he concluded. "They gave me that in the Emergency Room. Can you give me more of that? I know opioid addiction is awful, and sad to see how far off the Red Road these addicts have strayed – a bunch of scary, skinny, toothless and full of rage shadows are all that remains – but I think I can handle it..."

"What did you tell him?" April asked when I related the story that evening.

I said we'd try another non-opioid medication. That there were medicines that could help his pain without potentially triggering the urge to start drinking.

"How did he respond?"

He was willing to try it, but I could tell he was disappointed. He wanted what worked – what he knew would help him. It's hard to withhold medicines from my patients that way.

"How is this different from what you were doing at FQHC" she asked.

At FQHC I could get a patient like this to the Orthopedists. There weren't limitation on available funds. Here I can hardly get patients to Physical Therapy, because the waiting list is over a hundred patients long. Where there aren't the resources to help these people, it's like administering over a lot of grounded birds flailing about with broken wings.

And where withholding controlled substances is concerned, at FQHC I made those decisions based on urine drug screens – usually negative for prescribed narcotics, and positive for cocaine and heroin. It's not like here, where it's mostly a matter of trying to keep patients from falling back on alcoholism.

"Michael, you 'withheld' the medicine to avoid suffering," she said. "It's your job to decide what this patient really needed and what was best for him. He told you that he didn't want to go back to alcohol. You're just keeping him from going back on that road - A road he told you had 'ruined his life.'"

"I know it's hard on you, though," she concluded. "You always take on the most difficult tasks..."

It turned out the patient was a Veteran. When he told me, I called the VA, and arranged Orthopedic services there. Afterwards, I went to a Veterans group, and asked other Veterans to enlist in VA services.

"By getting specialty services through the VA," I said, "more is left in the Contract Health pot to help those who don't have other resources."

One Veterans stood and turned to the others.

"We got to do this guys," he said. "This is another way we help the vulnerable ones…"

CHAPTER EIGHTY-NINE

At the clinic I received a call that one of my patients was in the Emergency Room. Arriving there the ER staff pointed me to a young man in the procedure room. His hand was in a cast, and I didn't recognize him at first. Then, he smiled, and it struck me that this was the young inmate I'd met the other day.

"What happened?" I asked. "I thought you were going to Rehab?"

"I did," he said, shamefaced. "This morning, I was trying to reach my wife. The day before, we were talking, and she was being so supportive. But Rehab is for 90 days, and I started thinking she couldn't wait that long. So I called again. But when she didn't answer, I started feeling really down."

"I hate feeling that way," he continued. "I got so angry that I just wanted to hit something. I was outside and there was this tree. I had a feeling I would break my hand if I struck it. I said to myself, 'Don't do it. You're going to break your hand.' But I couldn't stop myself."

I nodded.

"I got my Indian name for an act of frustration," I said. "I was upset about having spent all night and the better part of the next day trying to justify a patient's admission to the hospital, only to come to find that the patient was better off getting his care somewhere else.

"I was so frustrated – That was the only day off I was going to get that week, and I'd just wasted it.

"I went to the Standing Elk Park to cool off. I took off my clothes and went walking headlong into the river – I just wanted to dunk my head.

"Then, just as I was about to get in, I tripped on something and heard a rattle; and when I looked back, saw a rattlesnake tumble into the water after me.

"I was scared, but the snake didn't come after me; fortunately, it just swam back to the shore. As it climbed up out of the river, I must have counted at least five rings on its tail.

"When I got back home, I told my neighbor about it; he said, 'From now on, your Indian name is 'Kicks the snake'."

The young man smiled and nodded.

"Kicks the snake," he repeated.

Then, his face lost expression.

"Have you ever felt so down that you just want to hurt yourself, Dr. Mike?" he asked.

As a matter of fact, I had. Some years ago, a friend asked if he could practice an alternative form of healing on me? I agreed, but, then, for no apparent reason, I experienced a feeling like my head was in a vice, and I couldn't breathe; and the feeling was so uncomfortable that – to endure it – I went about clenching my fists and digging my nails into my palms.

The patient quietly nodded.

"After I hit the tree," he continued, "it felt like my mind was clear again. I didn't feel any pain; instead, all of these thoughts came flooding back to me. They were memories from my childhood. I remembered being sexually abused. It was one of the teachers from the boarding school. Whenever I had to go, he would escort me into the bathroom. Then, he put Vaseline on my butt when I'd pull down my underwear.

"I remember crying. Why would he do that? I remember this guy teaching me to tie my shoes. How could he teach me to do that, and then be so evil?

"This went on for six months, until I finally told my mom. She went straight to the school. She left me outside the building, but I could still hear her screaming at the principal. There were some other teachers there, and I could hear what they were saying. I heard one of them say, 'How could you have a son like that?'

"I feel nauseous when I try to think about what happened. I try to see the good in everybody, but this morning I was seeing the bad. If I see the good, I could pull myself out of feeling down. With positive thoughts, you can go up.

"People do drugs because they're hurt and broken inside, and the drugs keep it so no one can see. But they're a trap. You have to be sober in order to feel comfortable and come out again.

"I just want to get my mind clear, so I can stop feeling down. I have really bad guilt about the things I've done. Things that have happened to me. I always feel like I'm shaking. I self-sabotage. I quit jobs. I have nightmares. I feel a lot of anger, but I don't act on it. Instead, I just walk away from things.

"I think the main thing is, I need is closure. I need to find closure for what happened when I was a kid..."

CHAPTER NINETY

While my clothes were drying at the laundromat, Ini and I walked into the nearby fields.

"The dog has to be on a leash," a woman called to me from the parking lot. "There are rules about that in town. You can't have your dog unleashed. This isn't the Reservation, you know."

I apologized and applied the leash, saying I rather regard my dog as a beloved companion that the Creator in His or Her infinite mercy felt kind enough to blessed me with. The woman looked on, disparagingly.

"They're like children," she said. "They need to be told what to do."

Ini wagged her tail and wiggled her whole body.

"That dog is really friendly," she said. "What did you say its name was?"

I told her, as well as the story behind it.

"That's really beautiful," she said.

Parting, I smiled; Ini does find a way to move beyond borders, I thought.

Then, coming upon some high brush, Ini stopped and stood at attention; then, before I could react, she lunged and dove into the brush, and this she did with such force that the leash was literally ripped from my hand. It turned out the source of movement was a bunny; it ran across the field, with Ini in hot pursuit...

"What was so interesting," I told April, "was that the first thought that went through my head that moment was 'Blackie'... - when that leash got yanked out of my hands - that night Blackie went after that other dog. The night that I lost her.

"All these years I've thought, 'If only I could have held onto that chain - if I just hadn't let go, I would have saved her.' But, today, that leash just broke right out of my hand. Ini jumped into that bush so quick and with such force that there was nothing I could do."

"I'm glad it gave you some closure, Michael," April said. "You can't save everyone. I know you want to, but sometimes it's beyond your control..."

CHAPTER NINETY-ONE

"I'd like to show you something, Dr. Mike," Somay said. "It's my art studio."

She led me to a large shed behind the house. Inside, large murals in different states of completion filled the work space, on tables and the walls.

"The murals are made from sand," she said. "I collect it from all over the Reservation."

There was rendering that looked like a view of the landscape seen from a low-flying plane; except that, although the farms and ranches appeared in an organized series of perfectly square plots of land, there seemed some sonic vibration uprooting them – like an energy wave unwilling to submit to the partitioned arrangement.

"The dominant culture wants things linear, but nature isn't like that," she said. "It's untamed. It's all beautiful, even the thorns."

In another mural of a river scene, the sand seem to capture light on the water, as though the mural were illuminated somehow.

"How do you get the quality of light?" I asked. "In paintings I always thought that was a matter of using white paint to create that effect. But you're achieving it with sand."

"I just learned it," she said. "By working with the sand and looking at the surroundings."

In a deep dark blue mural that of the Plains at twilight were the faint outlines of three wolves staring out, with a label next to it reading, 'Guardians.'

High on the wall hung a colorful rendering of a woman hugging an earthen globe. The woman appeared in a state of quiet joy and bliss, and, staring up at it, I thought of April and Somay.

Uchi Maka, I thought. Mother Earth.

On the floor was a large, intricate mural that Somay was currently working on. It seemed something of a self-portrait, showing an artist viewed from the back working in her studio. The artist had long, dark hair and wore a loose-fitting red blouse (the same as Somay), working on a canvas, ideas flowing from her, so to expand beyond the confines of the canvas; visions of fields with flowers and buffalo and rivers; but just beyond the studio's four walls was a world of suffering: people crawling about with broken bodies, replete with open wounds, dragging their limbs behind them; others cold without adequate firewood to keep them warm; thin and wasted without enough food to eat; searching through the waste and rubble of shattered buildings for nourishment and fuel. And, back in the studio, the floorboards supporting the artist were cracked and broken, sinking into the ground below, flooded by a distant dam.

"Is this what you're afraid of?" I asked.

"There's the world as it is and the world we're making," she responded. "We have to create the world – by putting out our intention."

"Dr. Mike, you came here with no ulterior motives," she continued. "Not really. It wasn't about advancing your career or having power. You wanted to help. You just wanted to be able to do what you were trained for. And what's happening on the Reservation has been beautiful, Dr. Mike. Word has spread – patients are coming to you. They're hearing about and wanting to see this new doctor, and turning out to see you. These are people who really avoid seeing somebody, as long as they can hold off, until they get to the point where they really have to. And you're the one they're going to go see. So you should take it as a pat on the shoulder. You started something new. You've created good change.

"But there's a part of you that isn't sure. It's holding you to the past. You're torn."

She looked away.

"'The powers that be' are always intent on keeping their own power," she said, "so it's never easy to effect change without bringing down the wrath of it all upon ourselves. That's why the world is in such a mess.

"It really is about intention. Your work of 'helping' is probably never going to be the straight ahead road that you envision. But we're being led into something even more powerful in its potential for bringing change.

"Maybe, you're past your 'barriers'? Maybe, the barriers were actually supporting you, and taking you to where you need to be? Maybe, if you don't keep crashing into barriers and trying to tear them away, you'll have the energy and freedom to seek the path where you can actually do more than you suspected you ever would be?

"There is magic and power in choosing one's experience - because seeing the Universe as always supportive allows one to see beyond the apparent limitations, and into new realms of possibility.

"You're a healer, Dr. Mike. Perhaps, you're being given new tools..."

CHAPTER NINETY-TWO

Returning to the Juvenile Detention Center, Orville sat in the front of the room and looked out at the young men who collected for his talk.

"You know, everything is easy today," he began. "With all this technology – cell phones, internet – you're never really far away. You can always talk to somebody.

"My mother's Indian name was Somay. Soloka is what we called the Crow Indians - for the blackbird that has the red spot on its wing. They were named after that. One day, I asked my mother, 'How come they call you Crow woman?' She said, 'Because I was born there.' I looked at her. 'How did that happen?'

"Well, my mother was born in 1893 – October. She said in 1893 my grandfather, who was a Chief, traveled to the Crow Agency, to make peace with the Crow Nation. She said he had a very simple message. At that time Reservations have been established all over the country. When he went there, he said, 'We're all fenced in now. And unless we work together, we will all die.'

"So, while he was meeting with the Crow leaders, my mother was born. And it was really interesting, because when he left, the Crow Nation gave him two herds of horses. One was all brown spotted horses. The other was all black – black spotted horses. And when they came back through Pine Ridge, they gave their relatives the brown spotted horses. The black spotted horses he brought here. That's what the Crow Nation did for us..."

CHAPTER NINETY-THREE

"When my mother was born," Orville continued, "in 1893, a lot of the traditions were still practiced. But they went underground, because they started enforcing the law in 1880. In 1880 the United States Congress passed a law outlawing all Indian spiritual practices across the country. You couldn't practice them without some kind of punishment. And that's why most of our people don't have any of the knowledge passed on."

"And they really enforced that law," he said, "in a very effective way. The missionaries – and it didn't matter which ones, they could belong to any church or denomination – when you died, if they knew you practiced any of the spiritual traditions – like praying with the pipe, or sweat lodge, or Sundance – they bury you outside the cemetery, and tell your family that you're burning in Hell."

He closed his eyes, and silently nodded.

"When you're five years old, and your favorite uncle is buried there, and they teach you how horrible Hell is, every day that you wake up, you're going to wonder, 'Is my uncle still burning?'... Because he prayed with a pipe.

"And you'll be afraid to pick up that pipe - because you might end up burning with him? So, it's a very effective way of giving young people the impression of what's going to happen if you practice any of this."

He opened his eyes again.

"If you ever go out east on Highway 29," he continued, "there is a little town called Canton. If you have time, stop in there. You'll see some graves. Most of them are unmarked. That's where they used to have an insane asylum for Indians. The ones who were institutionalized were medicine man, spiritual leaders, or anybody who practiced any of the ceremonies.

"In the records they write about how they brought in a young man, saying, 'He was insane - because he stood up on a hill, half naked, and he was talking to nobody.' The poor guy was doing a VisionQuest, and they said he was insane.

"So that kind of thing – and then the boarding schools – where they take you when you're five years old, and they punish you, for speaking your language.

"It was really hard. I was lucky. I didn't get into a boarding school system until I was sixteen. So, I could defend myself. But I saw little kids get really punished. And they learn to shut up, and not talk in their language.

"Sometimes we would sneak off, and visit in our language. Because if you're a fluent speaker, the English language is very hard to learn.

"I'm still learning. I tried to speak it all my life, and I'm still making mistakes. And there's a lot of words I don't understand. It's a hard language to learn – English."

"But these are the issues that we've come through the last hundred years or so," he said, "that forced your parents - your grandparents - to deny their Indian-ness..."

CHAPTER NINETY-FOUR

During the night I dreamt I was back in medical school. I was presenting to an instructor; the first presentation went well, as a described a patient who had cancer everywhere; but, for the next, I couldn't find my notes; then, when I did find them, I didn't seem familiar with what I was presenting, and the extent of his affliction left me uncomfortable and overwhelmed.

"I'm familiar with this patient," the instructor interrupted. "He was engaged in death games..."

In the afternoon Dr. Curtiz pulled me aside.

"Mike, I want to ask your help with something," he said. "There's someone I want you to meet."

Accompanying him to his examination room, an older, rugged looking native gentleman was sitting, and appeared strangely mute.

"Lyle here has throat cancer," Curtiz said. "We found it because he was complaining of swallowing problems and being hoarse. It's a particularly aggressive cancer... Undifferentiated squamous cell carcinoma, metastatic to the ribs, lungs, liver and kidneys. He's had chemotherapy and just finished radiation, but things aren't getting any better. Despite the feeding tube, he's losing weight, doesn't feel right and can hardly think straight."

Lyle wore a vacant expression, as though he weren't sure where he was and appeared disoriented.

"I think that it's time to call it quits," Curtiz said. "It's time to bring him in. I explained to him that I think it's time."

"Mike, I think it's about time that I entrusted Lyle to your care," he continued. "You know a lot more about cancer than I do. I'm just an old family practice doc. It's time for you to take over. Please write admitting orders and take over Lyle's treatment... I just think that you're the man to do it. I think you should take over this case..."

That evening I talked with April.

"I'm surprised he'd hand a patient over that way?" I said. "In the patient's hour of greatest need?"

"Well, maybe he realizes his limitations," she responded, "and he meant it when he said that you were the best person to take over this patient's care..."

CHAPTER NINETY-FIVE

Around midnight a call came from the hospital.

"Mr. Lyle removed his IV and spilled blood all over the floor," the charge nurse said. "Then, he walked around half-naked through the corridor until he finally sat on a commode that belonged to another patient in a different room..."

Arriving on the ward, I helped the nurses guide Lyle back to his room. Blood work showed particularly high levels of calcium.

"The cancer in his bones is driving up the calcium in his bloodstream," I told the pharmacist. "That calcium is going to his brain and making it difficult for him to think straight. I'm ordering a medication to lower his calcium levels. Can you prepare it?"

The pharmacist was familiar with Lyle, and immediately came to the hospital.

"Oh, yeah, Lyle was really robust," he said. "He was always smiling. Just one of these really positive, upbeat kind of guys. I could tell something was wrong when I saw him in the waiting room today and he wasn't smiling. He must be in a lot of pain."

Indeed, he was receiving narcotics at high dose.

"Lyle is pretty stoic," the pharmacist emphasized. "I think it comes from all those years of Sundancing. That's a very painful and difficult ritual. He can tolerate a lot of pain. If he complains about something, it means that the pain is off the rector scale... Yeah, off the charts..."

CHAPTER NINETY-SIX

Rounding the following morning, the charge nurse greeted me, smiling.

"What did you do, Doc?" she said. "Lyle is like a different person. He's so much more with it than he was before. Was it all just that calcium? I wish someone would have fixed that sooner…"

Nevertheless, a repeat of calcium showed his levels were still high, and that coupled with narcotics put him at risk for cardiac arrest.

"Lyle, if your heart should stop beating," I said, "would you want us to try to bring you back?"

He looked at me unsure, shrugged his shoulders, and indicated at his throat that he was unable to speak. When he gestured to my clipboard, I handed it to him. He wrote slow and deliberately.

I would like to be brought back. But no extreme measures. I don't want to be kept alive by machines.

I nodded.

"If resuscitation were necessary," I said, "then, at least for a time and perhaps the rest of your life, a machine might have to breathe for you. How do you feel about that?"

He went back to writing on the pad.

No one has ever talked about this before. I can't decide. I'll tell you in the morning…

CHAPTER NINETY-SEVEN

Sitting at the nurses station reviewing charts, I had the distinct feeling of being watched. Looking up, Ryan, Orville and Somay were standing over me.

"Sir, can I get a hamburger and fries?" Ryan said, leaning forward on the counter.

The nurses laughed.

"I did that in a library one time," Ryan continued. "The librarian said, 'Sir, this is a library. You have to speak quietly.' So I bent down like this and whispered, 'Can I get a hamburger and fries?'"

I led them to Lyle's room. At the doorway, Orville smiled wide as he approached his ill friend. Somay stayed behind with me.

"Dad's known Lyle for a long time," she confided. "For years Lyle and dad would Sundance side-by-side."

She turned to me.

"Have you been to dad's Sundance?" she asked.

I nodded, saying I'd talked about it recently with a patient, and the experience that led the patient to say I'd been touched by a spirit helper.

"You had," she said. "You should dance."

I don't think so, I said. I don't think I really understand it.

"It's how you give back after asking for something," she said. "Like when you make a prayer for someone to get better. In exchange, you dance."

She hesitated.

"I told you I had meningitis," she said. "I think I was six. Maybe, I was older - eight or nine. Anyway, they did a lumbar puncture on me. The first time they said the results were inconclusive, so they had to do it again. When they did the second one, it was really painful, and there was some complication, so, afterwards, I couldn't move my legs. Then, I couldn't move my arms. And I couldn't pee.

"The doctors told my mom and dad that I wasn't going to get better. They told them that I was going to die… That's what they actually said - that I was 'going to die.'

"So my parents said, 'If she's going to die, then we want to take her home, so that she could die surrounded by family.'

"They brought me home and my dad invited healers come from all over the Reservation to come and work on me. They took me in the sweat lodge and prayed over me. It didn't seem like I was getting any better, but they kept trying.

"Dad noticed that I was growing hair on my arms. He went to the hospital and asked my doctor. The doctor said it was because they had given me steroids in the hospital. When dad asked why he hadn't told him before that or explained the side effects or asked for his permission, the doctor just said it was because he knew I was going to die.

"One day, my mom sat me on the toilet. They kept on putting me there to pee, even though they were cath-ing me, and I was in diapers all the time because I had no control of it. But this time, I felt like I could do it. When I started to pee, I called to my mom. She was so happy that she lifted me up, and hugged me, and laughed, and started crying.

"After that, I had to learn to walk again. I had to learn to run. It was really hard.

"That's when dad began Sundancing. He hadn't Sundanced before that. He felt like this was what he had to do to offer thanks to the Creator - so I'd keep getting well. That's where he met Lyle. Lyle was Sundancing, too. He helped dad. Later, he helped me."

She paused.

"My mother was involved in a car accident," she continued. "Her skull was cracked, and the doctor said that she wouldn't be able to see with one of her eyes, and she'd be paralyzed on her left side.

"So I prayed that she would get well and was told that she would get better, but that I had to dance.

"So I danced, and when we got mother home, her sight got better and she was able to move her left side.
"I danced every season until one year my mom told me that she didn't want me to dance anymore – she was ready to go. So I didn't dance that season, and later that year she died. Before that, I danced for ten years…"

CHAPTER NINETY-EIGHT

"Is he going to get better when you lower his calcium?" April asked.

Only symptomatically, I said. His condition is still terminal.

"So his cancer has advanced to a point that it can't be treated?" she said.

Yes. I'd spoken with his oncologist; he informed me that Lyle had a very aggressive form of cancer, and previous treatment for it had been purely palliative.

"How long do you think he has?" she asked. "Do you see him at the hospital for weeks, days, months?"

I didn't know.

"I keep adjusting his morphine for pain control," I said. "Increasing his IV fluids to get rid of high calcium in this blood stream."

"What would you like to see for this guy?" she asked.

I'd like to see him go out with the coming Sundance, I said.

"Well, see it as an opportunity," she responded, enthusiastically. "See it as Dr. Curtiz handing you someone who many in the community care about. Now, you can take over and oversee the last stage of his life. You can say, 'I'm taking care of someone that Orville and Somay really care about. I'm glad he ended up in my lap...'"

CHAPTER NINETY-NINE

At Morning Report I announced that Lyle's condition was stable. "He's probably ready for discharge to hospice," I said.

Within the room there was a collective silence, and among the members of the hospital staff, it seemed that all heads turned in the direction of Dr. Curtiz, who sat with his gaze directed downward.

"There is no hospice here, Mike," Curtiz said. "We have no way to provide assistance to terminal patients out in the community."

I looked at him, confused. What's the usual protocol for caring for terminally ill patients? I asked.

"Usually, those services are provided in the hospital," he responded...

"It's kind of tricky – your doing hospice care," April commented. "You're being put in an awkward situation... Because you're not a hospice doc – Your job is to keep people alive..."

CHAPTER ONE HUNDRED

On a trail near the medical complex, Ini and I walked in the fields. Not far, a couple walked ahead. They looked so young, and yet had two children in tow. I thought about the possibility of a peaceful life. Perhaps, these two ahead were living such an existence? Perhaps, I could, too? Here. Just enjoying life. Enjoying the experience. Enjoying each other.

"That's what life is all about..."

The image of a recurring dream from childhood entered my head; a man – perhaps, an older version of my young self - walked along a dusty road; two young children – a boy and a girl - run towards him; he hoists the girl on his shoulders; the boy he takes by the hand; they continue walking; in the distance a house appears; a dark haired woman stands outside at the patio by the doorway; she greets him with a kiss.

Perhaps, we could have children? I thought. And just live. Stay here on the Reservation – away from the crowds and cities. Live naturally as we were meant to, and keep the rest of the world outside?

My reverie was interrupted by the feeling of being nudged at my leg. Looking down Ini was gazing up at me, having dropped the ball at my feet. I collected the ball and walked towards the house.

Passing the basketball court in the park near my home, there were a couple of little boys playing. I was watching the boys when out of nowhere, two compact, little dogs came charging and chasing after Ini. I pulled Ini away, but the small dogs kept pursuing her. The boys on the basketball court stopped their game and called and ran after the small dogs.

"They're pit bulls," the older boy said. "We asked our mom for a leash, but she said she didn't want to leash them. She wanted to let them run free."

Relentlessly, the smaller dogs kept after Ini; the boys chased after them, but the dogs just scattered only to regroup and go after Ini again. Then, the smaller boy slid and scraped his knee.

"Are you alright?" I asked.

He grimaced and I went to help him. Still, the small dogs nipped at Ini. Finally, I lifted Ini and carried her away...

"You took control of the situation," April said. "Because you got her out of there."

But I kept thinking about the two boys.

"Yeah, ridiculous," she said. "In the park by themselves watching over free range dogs that do not listen to voice control."

My mind flashed to my brother and me the night that we were alone and Blackie broke from the chain; the look of the smaller boy who hurt his knee, and the thought of my brother as he lifted Foxy – his shirt all bloody.

"Foxy went into Blackie's territory," April said. "If you had had a fence, Foxy wouldn't have been able to come in. But the neighbors could have had a fence, too. They didn't build a fence, either."

No, our neighbors had had a fence. It was by choice that the neighbors let Foxy roam the neighborhood.

"They let the dog run around all the time!?" April responded.

Yes, I said. I'd always put the blame on Blackie for that night that he went after Foxy. Now, for the first time, it occurred to me that it wasn't completely Blackie's fault.

And my brother and I had been little different than the two boys tonight. I'd known something of the same chaos as these boys. Like them I hadn't had someone there to help me, and, as a result, been forced to give up something I loved...

CHAPTER ONE HUNDRED AND ONE

At 2 AM I was awoke by a call from the hospital.

"Doctor, your patient Lyle is having problems breathing," the charge nurse said. "We've given him oxygen, but it isn't helping. He was hardly able to get up when friends visited. When he tried to get up, he fell back in bed."

Making my way to the hospital, a strong wind blew. In the moonlight the high grass rippled like waves in the ocean.

Entering the ward it seemed as dark and still as it was outside. Even the heart monitors seemed oddly silent as they continued their tracings.

Entering Lyle's room, he lay still in bed. His hospital gown was soaked with sweat and he felt warm to the touch. His heart was beating fast and pounding; his breath sounds diminished on the right side.

"He's septic," I said. "Probably pneumonia."

"Should we transfer him to another hospital?" the nurse asked.

I shook my head. The nearest facility was three hours away, and make it difficult for friends and family to visit.

"Let's do what we can for him here," I said.

We started IV antibiotics and high-flow oxygen. A radiology tech performed a chest x-ray, and I walked downstairs to view it on the lightbox. It showed a large focus of pneumonia in the right lung. I ordered breathing treatments each hour and stayed with Lyle through the night...

"Curtiz knew what he was doing when he passed the patient on to you," April said. "Wow, so what are you going to do?"

If he makes it, we'll keep talking. Lyle still hadn't signed a DNR order, so there was nothing to do except keep working to pull him through.

At about 8 AM Somay and Wesley arrived at the room. Lyle still lay unconscious.

"We've done everything we could," I said, "but it looks like the cancer is getting the best of him."

Somay nodded, then opened her purse and took out some photographs.

"I wanted to show you this," she said. "This is what Lyle looked like last October, just after the last Sundance."

In the photo Lyle stood looking stoic between a smiling Orville and Somay. He appeared robust in Lakota regalia, wearing a hair pipe breastplate over his broad chest, with leather bands strapped around muscular biceps. Looking back to the figure in the bed – Body wasted, features sunken, breathing labored, it seemed little remained except the shell of what he'd been...

CHAPTER ONE HUNDRED AND TWO

Returning to Lyle's room, Somay sat embroidering a quilt, while Wesley lay asleep in the cot next to her.

"Administration was pretty quick to let Somay have her sewing machine here," the charge nurse said. "It usually takes an act of Congress to make any changes in policy here. But considering the circumstances, they didn't give Somay much trouble."

"I think that Lyle was getting a little uncomfortable when Wesley was running all over the room," Somay said. "He was just being a typical kid. He's going to want to explore places and run here and there."

Somay commented that Lyle had awoken and seemed like he was responding to the medication.

"Lyle is definitely getting better, though he still has his moments when he's kind of out of it," she said. "The nurse told me that this morning when Lyle woke up, he asked for his walker. 'Where are you planning on going, Lyle?' she asked him. 'I'm going to head over to Orville's camp for some oatmeal this morning.' That's what he used to do every year when we'd all Sundance together. He'd come down to our camp, and we'd share some oatmeal..."

"He's at the Sundance, which is just what you wanted for him," April said. "Where you wanted him to be..."

CHAPTER ONE HUNDRED AND THREE

Making rounds, Lyle was sitting up in bed. When I asked how he was doing, he motioned for my notepad.

Fine. How are you?

I lifted my brow.

Well, to be truthful, I said, I've had a rather frustrating day.

The gaunt and dying man looked at me concerned, and motioned for the notepad again.

What happened?

My brother called, wanting me to prescribe him some medication. He lives in Los Angeles, and I'd told him I didn't feel comfortable prescribing over the phone. He didn't take that well, and hung up the phone. Lyle nodded.

What does your brother do?

He's a lawyer, but he mostly surfs. He lives with my mom.

I guess he's the one who won the bet.

Looking back, he was smiling with a certain gleam in his eye. I smiled, too. Then, he went back to writing.

My brother came and visited me today. I don't think he understands how sick I am. I think he didn't want to think about it. But now I think he knows.

"Are you close?" I asked.

We're brothers. You know how that is.

I nodded in agreement.

Better not to hold grudges. It just gets in the way.

My attempt to nod ended in a sideways motion.

Better we should live like dogs, and spend every moment loving each other. They can because from the start they know they won't live long and need to do what's important...

CHAPTER ONE HUNDRED AND FOUR

Having reviewed Lyle's latest lab findings, I went to his room to discuss further treatment options.

"Your white blood cell count suggests the infection in your lungs has cleared," I said. "Now, we need to work on better pain control and titrate the morphine you require."

Somay and Orville were standing nearby; between the three, there seemed a quiet understanding for which I had been yet to be included.

"Lyle doesn't want any more treatment," Somay said. "Today, Lyle told dad that he didn't want to wake up again and to pray that the next time he closed his eyes he wouldn't open them again."

I looked at them, surprised. Lyle nodded.

"He's requesting that IV fluids and antibiotics be stopped," she continued.

I bowed my head and stepped back.

"Then, I'll respect your wishes," I said. "Should you reconsider, please let me know..."

CHAPTER ONE HUNDRED AND FIVE

"Were you really so surprised by his decision?" April asked. "From the beginning you told me that his case was terminal."

I guess I'd gotten used to being there for him, I responded. For the past weeks I've attended him every day without fail. Even when I could have asked Dr. Curtiz to cover for me, I hadn't.

"Mike, you're going to be leaving there sooner or later," she said. "There's only a few months left on your NHSC obligation. Where are things with plans for coming back here?"

I hadn't made any.

"Why not, Mike?" she responded, disappointed. "What are you waiting for?"

There's no coming back for me, I said. Not after FQHC. We'd already been down that road. There wasn't a clinic or health center that would touch me. This was the only place that would have me.

"Mike, I watched you slug it out before," she said. "After you were let go by FQHC, you kept on sending out those resumes and applying for those jobs and dealing with all the credentialing requirements and blah, blah, blah.

"You had a disagreeable CEO and weakling Clinical Director. And you had to deal with that.

"And you wanted to stay, but they forced you out. So, you got up in the morning, you put on your clothes, and you did those job interviews. And you came home totally drained, unappreciated by higher ups – but very appreciated by lower ups. And you got up that next morning and you went at again until you got it done. You got a position at the Indian Reservation where you had friends. You're on your way to getting your NHSC commitment cleared. And how did you get all of that done? By getting up in the morning, putting one foot in front of the other, until you went to sleep, and got up the next morning, and did the same thing until it was done.

"And that's a very valuable skill, and I really, really respect you for that. I wish I had known that about you when we first got married. I think I would have been a lot less scared. And I think that whole experience would have been a lot better for both of us if I had known that about you.

"But I didn't know that about you. I had to learn it. If I had realized the inner strength you have, and the fact that you just keep on going until you find a solution, then I wouldn't have been as scared as I was.

"Not everybody gets up. Some people face adversity, and they give up. They don't have that inner energizer bunny that tells them, 'Get up and keep going. And go to sleep, and get up, and keep going. Until you get somewhere.' And every morning, you just get up and just keep going. Doesn't matter how many times somebody slaps you down, or how hopeless it looks. You just get up the next day, and keep going.

"Obviously, I'm not as strong as you are. I don't think I believe in myself the same way you believe in yourself..."

"You have it in you to do the same thing with this next challenge," she concluded. "And then it will be done, and you can move on – knowing that you've done everything you could to make things better. You can do anything you want..."

Job Announcement:
Deputy Director, Office of Clinical and Preventive Services (OCPS)
Description: Provide leadership to improve and promote wellness for
American Indian and Alaska Native (AI/AN) people overseeing the
following programs:

- *Division of Behavioral Health (DBH)*
- *Division of Diabetes Treatment and Prevention (DDTP)*
- *Division of Nursing Services (DNS)*
- *Division of Oral Health (DOH)*
- *Improving Patient Care (IPC)*
- *Risk Management (RM)...*

CHAPTER ONE HUNDRED AND SIX

The hospital pharmacist pulled me aside.

"Hey, Dr. Mike, I was thinking about you while I was looking on the IHS website," he said. "They have an opening for an administrator at Headquarters… Deputy Director for the Office of Clinical and Preventive Services. OCPS oversees some of the most important Departments in Indian health. We're talking Diabetes, Risk Management, Behavioral Health. You'd have a platform to make a whole lot more changes than the ones you're currently looking into with the VA."

"I just think you'd be a natural for it," he continued. "I see you as a 'systems' guy. Your organizational talents are wasted here. I just think you'd be doing a lot more good for people there than what you can do for them here. Would hate to lose you here, but this might be an opportunity that comes around only once…"

"Yeah, I can see you in that position," April said. "I think that's something for you. Having a voice in how things are done there."

How would I do that? I said. I had no experience in policy making.

"You'll learn, Mike," she said. "You have a PhD in cancer. You have a track record for succeeding at anything you put your mind to."

My cancer vaccine days are behind me, I said. I left because I wanted to care for others the way they cared for me. I'm a doctor now. I want to keep working as a physician.

"In South Dakota?!" she responded. "Because the way things are, a doctor like you can only work in exile. Is that what you want? For you? For your fellow physicians? So they can be fired for no reason other than serving as a moral, ethical physician to their patients and communities, and then not be able to find work, or have

200

to move away from their wives and families, even when their wives are sick and undergoing treatment for cancer? Is that what you want? For you? For your fellow physician? Because that's what there is. And it needs to be changed. And no one knows that better than you.

"And I know you love your Clinical Director there – and he loves you. But there's more out there for you, Mike. You might be able to change all those things you want to. If you're willing to get your head out of the sand and fight for it..."

Application: Deputy Director, Office of Clinical and Preventive Services. Please prepare a written statement addressing each of the following:

(1) Demonstrate substantial knowledge of the Federal Health Care Delivery Systems (rural and urban).

(2) Demonstrate experience evaluating policy options, forecasting costs, benefits and long-term results.

(3) Demonstrate experience and ability in formulating, implementing and evaluating high-impact policies, programs and projects and advising senior executives of a large organization on options or resolving problems caused by existing or proposed policies or conditions.

(4) Demonstrate experience and working knowledge of disseminating information to customers and the general public.

(5) Demonstrate progressive experience in effectively managing a comprehensive and complex interdisciplinary health program target to serve the underserved and underprivileged...

CHAPTER ONE HUNDRED AND SEVEN

At the invitation of IHS Headquarters I flew to Washington, DC to interview for the Deputy Director position. The passenger seated next to me was a man of considerable girth that continually spilled into my space. As I sat reviewing materials, I noticed my neighbor peering over my shoulder.

"The handouts this country gives to Indians is the worst thing next to welfare," he declared loudly to his wife on the other side. "That should be the first entitlement the government gets rid of."

At the time I stayed quiet. Later, I engaged him in conversation.

"So, what do you do for a living?" I asked.

"I own a hotel," he responded, proudly.

"Oh, so you make money renting rooms to people," I responded. "You wonder if native peoples would need all these 'handouts' and 'entitlements' if they could have rented their land to the rest of us?"

The man went silent, and uttered not another word for the rest of the flight. When the plane landed, he pushed past me without a word, as he and his wife hastily departed...

CHAPTER ONE HUNDRED AND EIGHT

Arriving at IHS Headquarters I was escorted to a conference room on the top floor of the building. Waiting, I stood gazing out at the DC skyline through the large plate glass windows that entirely went around the room. Then, like clockwork, the door opened at the designated hour for the interview, and the Chief Medical Officer glided in.

"So, I see you've spent time working in the field," she said. "What makes you interested in a job at Headquarters?"

My heart beats for the IHS, I responded. Working in the IHS has given me the opportunity to realize my goal of striving to help address the most pressing medical challenge facing the nation: making healthcare affordable, and, at the same time, assuring proper patient care. It's my intent to take what I've learned in the field and apply it to policy making.

"What do you feel you could bring to the position?"

First-hand experience working in the private sector, and an appreciation for the federal system, particularly the IHS, which does the most with the least, and offers a model to keep national healthcare afloat, as opposed to privately-owned systems, which threaten to sink the ship national healthcare. Just before joining the IHS I worked at a privately owned federally qualified health center, and observed a number of practices that concerned me. These practices included the prescribing of controlled substances without proper oversight. It was my feeling that these practices placed patients and the community at risk of addiction. In contrast, my experience in the Indian Health Service has been entirely different, supporting a responsible approach to treating patients with controlled substances.

"Tell me about your path through medicine?"

I suppose it began in college; as an undergraduate I studied tumor specific antibodies to treat patients with lymphoma. The summer before medical school I worked at the Weizmann Institute of Science in Rehovot, Israel, defining the molecular mechanisms of the p53 oncogene, which is mutated in a majority of human cancers. As a Howard Hughes scholar in medical school, I went to National Institutes of Health, and took the lead in developing a vaccine for cancer that targeted p53 mutations, which won FDA approval for clinical trials in patients with advanced malignancies.

"It sounds like you did a lot of research. What made you want to go into primary care?"

I hurt my leg while working on the cancer vaccine. I was in constant pain, and prescribed all manner of medications; most just caused side effects, and what really helped me was striking up relationships with fellow patients suffering from similar conditions as me; they were the ones who really got me better, and I made a promise that after I finished my PhD, I'd help others the way they helped me. Still, it's just part of me to see the bigger picture, and want to effect larger change.

"Has that ever translated into transformative system change?"

My work at a rural West Tennessee medical center was said to have ushered in a hospitalist program; I'd received commendations from the Tennessee Health Department for my part in transforming a health center rated the worst in the state to a 'model of excellence'; working with Native Veterans on the Reservation, I'd spearheaded efforts to integrate care between the IHS and VA.

"Do you have experience or expertise in Mental Health?"

Three years ago I'd been present on the Reservation during the 2010 Memorial Day suicide cluster. Afterwards, I assisted in community-based suicide prevention programs that brought native healers from all over the Northern Plains to help at risk children. There hadn't been a suicide cluster since.

"Do you have any ideas for making changes on the Reservations?"

Freud said the two most vital parts to the health of a person – mental, physical and spiritual – were love and work. Unemployment on the Reservation is 80-90%, and I've wondered how that affects the health of the people on the Reservation? My father sits on a number of Boards of Directors for industry. When I shared my concerns about work on the Reservation with him, he's responded by quoting the Wall Street Journal, saying how it's getting more and more expensive to get things from China, and they're no longer the low cost producer in the world that they were. Now, hundreds and hundreds of people are needed to do this work, and saying if it was up to him, he'd be looking for low cost labor, and if there was a ready work force, then putting it on a Reservation where he imagined there was the possibility of all kinds of tax breaks and not paying property taxes, then it might be a good deal, and there were advantages to that. I'd shared these ideas with tribal leaders, and they'd responded with support...

...Mike is trustworthy, accountable and transparent. He supports tactics that best ensure safe and sound medical practices. He contributes to quality care through staff education and training; building a competent workforce that is capable of achieving high standards within the Agency. He is mindful of the budget limitations and work towards maximizing efforts at minimal costs to achieve high Government Performance and Results Act scores. He has represented the Area in the National Pharmacy & Therapeutics Committee and volunteered to participate in physician recruitment efforts. His performance is OUTSTANDING! He is an exceptional asset to the Indian Health Service and should be considered for positions of leadership within our organization...
James Curtiz MD...

CHAPTER ONE HUNDRED AND NINE

Returning from DC I resumed work at the hospital. Making rounds Orville was in Lyle's room, sitting beside his old friend.

"You're just in time, Doc," Orville said, smiling broadly. "I invited the regulars from the Sweat to come and make a ceremony here for Lyle."

He showed me some freshly cut sage.

"I picked it from the Sundance grounds," he said. "We'll use it to purify the room?"

I asked if he planned to burn it.

"Yeah, sure, Doc," he responded.

I shook my head.

It's against hospital policy, I said. It's not permitted.

He looked at me, confused.

"But, Dr. Mike, it's just some sage," he said.

It could set off the fire alarms and sprinkler system in the hospital, I said. If the curtains were to catch on fire, it might be that the hospital would have to be evacuated, and put lives at risk. There were patients on the ward with breathing problems, and the burning of sage could potentially exacerbate their condition.

Orville gazed at Lyle.

"I'm sorry," I concluded. "I can't sanction it…"

CHAPTER ONE HUNDRED AND TEN

Within an hour of leaving the ward, a call came from the charge nurse.

"Lyle says he's going home," she said. "He's getting ready to leave."

I hurried back. Entering the room Lyle was already dressed, and packing the remainder of his belongings.

"Whoa, whoa, whoa," I said. "Wait. Is this because of what I said about the ceremony?"

But Lyle just continued silently moving back and forth between the dresser and a small suitcase on the bed.

"Please don't go," I said. "You won't have the same level of care at home. You won't have the same services available to you to control your pain. The past days you've been requiring increased doses of morphine. You won't have the pain pump with you. Please. Please stay."

Lyle sat heavily on the bed, then motioned for my pen and notepad, and, slowly and methodically, began to write.

I'll be fine, he wrote in his slow, deliberate fashion. My brother will take care of me.

I shook my head, speechless. He looked at me, raised a hand to my shoulder and then went back to writing. he wrote on the pad.

This has all been my fault, doctor. Orville and Somay wouldn't tell you, but I was an alcoholic. Whenever I felt bad, I would drink. I lived that way for years.

Finally, I had enough and tried to go sober. When I felt bad about things and had the urge to drink, I would go to a friends or ceremony and talk and keep on moving, trying to stay away from the bottle, for another day, another hour, until now it's been two years that I've been sober.

Sitting beside him, I recalled the last time I'd tried to visit my uncle; I'd called and said I was passing through, and asked if I could stop by? He'd said he was busy helping his daughter pack her things to go back to college; I offered to help, but he told me, "Keep driving."

My mistake, I reflected. I guess I thought we were family.

I did this to me, Clayton continued. I know that.

I shook my head. No, I thought. Don't leave. You're among friends… family.

Thank you for taking care of me. You're a good doctor. I appreciate everything you done…

CHAPTER ONE HUNDRED AND ELEVEN

April had arranged a trip to Yellowstone. Meeting her at the airport, she excitedly ran through our planned itinerary.

"For the first night I got us a hotel in the Park at the lake," she said. "After that, we'll circle around to east end of the Park, where they have all that interesting geology. That's what I want to see, but I'm afraid you'll just think they're a lot of smelly geysers and sulfur pits, so I we'll go over there first. I booked us a room where they said you could actually see Old Faithful out the window. After that, we'll head to the west end of the park. That's where they have most of the buffalo herds. I figured you'd like that the most, so I saved it for last. Did you board Ini in a kennel?"

No, I left her with Somay; she and Wesley will look after her.

At the baggage carousel I stood, quiet

"Is something the matter, Mike?" she asked.

I'd been thinking about Lyle.

"Well, do you want to go back?" she asked.

No, I said. He'd made his decision. He has a right to do things his way.

"But maybe you could help?" she said.

I shook my head.

I'd signed out with Dr. Curtiz, I said. If Lyle had a problem, Curtiz would be there to help.

Collecting her bags, we went to the car, and set off for the Yellowstone; then, not an hour into our trip, a call came from an oddly familiar number with Montana area code?

"Hello, Dr. Mike. This is Frank Lightning. Are you surprised to hear from me?... I understand you came back here."

Before that moment, I hadn't heard or spoken with him in over two years.

"I want to invite you to the Reservation where I live," he said. "Here in Lame Deer. I want to show you something. Are you interested?"

Yes, I said, but I'm with my wife, and we're on our way to Yellowstone.

"The Yellowstone isn't far," he said. "You can stop by and then be on your way..."

"Who was that?" April asked.

"That was Frank," I said. "The traditional horse expert I met the first time I came here. He invited us to visit him... In Montana where he lives."

I hesitated.

"He said it was on the way," I continued, sheepishly. "Would you mind taking a little detour?..."

CHAPTER ONE HUNDRED AND TWELVE

Arriving at Frank's, April had been behind the wheel.

"What besides driving this guy all around do you do?" Frank said half-jokingly.

"I'm an art conservator," April responded.

"April worked at the National Museum of the American Indian," I inserted. "She was the one who got me interested in native culture and traditions. If it wasn't for her, we probably would have never met."

Frank nodded, looking at her as though unsure, and studying her.

"Why do you think you stand like that?" he asked, indicating her hunched shoulders.

I reflexively turned and looked at April, then back at Frank.

That's an odd question, I thought.

But April appeared unfazed.

"When I was in school," she responded, "I went through puberty and developed breasts earlier than the other girls in my class. Because of that, I was teased. So I kept my shoulders hunched, so that I could hide them, and the others wouldn't tease me as much."

"Shame," Frank responded. "Shame is not a feeling unknown to my people. Shame for our ways. Shame for our dark skin. And for those reasons, we were taken away from our loved ones, and sent to boarding schools, made to feel ashamed of our language. Made to feel ashamed of our traditions. Made to feel ashamed of our dark skin. We were made to feel ashamed of ourselves. And this shame still exists in our culture, and needs to be reconciled, just like the shame in your shoulders.

"Where alcohol is concerned, this is a way that was given to our people by the whites to cope with our shame. The problem is, it erodes the Indian soul. It takes from the Indian, and leaves us with nothing but an empty shell. That's what years of drinking does, and that's why it needs to be stopped in our population. We just do not have the genes for it. That's why the alcohol affects us more than the whites."

"The same is true of carbohydrates," he added. "We just don't have the means to break down the alcohol and carbohydrates the way that the whites do."

Frank nodded.

"Tomorrow, I will take you to the very ground where a hundred years ago the four holders of the White Buffalo Calf Woman's Sacred Pipe came together in the Sundance ceremony where Sitting Bull had his vision for what he needed to defeat the whites and protect and preserve his people from the armies that were coming to annihilate them," he said. "I will take you there tomorrow. Be ready. Because after this, you're going to receive communications from the spirits, and your life will not be the same..."

CHAPTER ONE HUNDRED AND THIRTEEN

"Before I take you to this place," Frank continued, "tonight, we'll do a Sweat. In the sweat lodge I bring people in and take them through the rebirthing process, so that they can learn how to bond and feel love and love their children. That's what we have to do to give our people back that part of their lives that was taken away from them – by the boarding schools, by the institutionalization that they've known all their lives, and the love that was replaced by drink."

Frank left the room. April turned.

"Mike, you know why you bond with these people, don't you?" she said. "It's because you suffer similar to the way they do... Your grandmother was an orphan. She didn't know how to bond with your mother. Your mother didn't feel loved by her. And she didn't know how to bond with you. That's the same kind of difficulty that these people have been living with and are now trying to heal. That's why you resonate with them so much..."

CHAPTER ONE HUNDRED AND FOURTEEN

No white person or persons shall be permitted to settle upon or occupy any portion of the territory, or without the consent of the Indians to pass through the same.
~ The Treaty of Laramie, 1868

Driving to the sacred site, Frank turned.

"Doctor, what comes into your mind when I ask you, 'What's not for sale?'" he said.

I shook my head.

My principles, I responded. The people I hold dear.

"To an Indian, it's the Black Hills," he said. "The Black Hills are not for sale. Because they're *holy.*"

"We fought for that land. Chief Red Cloud waged a war. It was the only time that the US military had been successfully defeated. It was to preserve our people's way of life and to keep that land holy.

"In 1868 the United States concluded the Red Cloud War by agreeing to the Treaty of Laramie, which effectively gave Indians the Black Hills.

"But gold was reported in the Black Hills, and in direct violation of the Treaty of Laramie, Custer and the 7th Cavalry were sent to validate these claims. Their expedition confirmed the presence of gold and a flood of white speculators began mining the area.

"The United States' government sent agents to buy the Black Hills. When they were told that they were holy and not for sale, they sent Custer to make war against the Lakota and the Cheyenne and Arapaho who were camped there. Native peoples on their lands, following the herds of buffalo, and providing for their people.

"At the battle of Little Bighorn when the cavalry came over the hill, they saw tipis that stretched for eleven miles. They knew that in those tipis were not just warriors – this was a community of men, women and children. And yet they rode right into that community without warning – to kill them.

"And this offends me because that never happened in any of the other wars fought in this country. That kind of warfare was never done anywhere else. Not in Europe. Not in the American Revolution. Not even in the Civil War. Battles were fought on battlefields. Women and children were evacuated.

"It's because to them, these weren't people. Indians weren't human. Their goal was to exterminate them.

"They were families, with old people and babies. There were little girls playing with dolls, and little boys who were just learning to walk. And the soldiers were sent to attack them and kill them all.

"It was done because they were Indian. We were the first people on this continent. And because of that, we had to be removed and done away with.

"And when my great-grandfather took to his horse, it was to protect his wife, his child, his community. And he fought and died protecting them. Not far from this ground.

"Custer had been warned. After he slaughtered innocent Cheyenne elders, women and children at the Washita River, our Chiefs decided to take pity on him, and forgive him, and invited him to their ceremonies, and passed him the sacred pipe to smoke. After Custer smoked, the Chiefs told him, 'Take those ashes from the pipe and put them on the ground.' He didn't know. He didn't ask, 'What for?' He just did it. Then, they said, 'Now, with your heel, bury those ashes into the earth.' And he did this, too. 'Now we are brothers,' the Chiefs said. 'But if you double cross us again, that will be you in the ash, and it will be of your own making.'…"

CHAPTER ONE HUNDRED AND FIFTEEN

We traversed a stone canyon with sedimentary layers of white, red, yellow and black.

"You see these," Frank said. "Do you recognize what colors they are?"

I said they were the sacred colors of the Lakota and Cheyenne people.

"They're the colors of the earth," he responded. "These are the colors of the medicine wheel. It tells us that we are all connected. It teaches us balance. It helps us get out of being unbalanced. It teaches us common sense, and gets us out of just linear ways of thinking and helps us to be spirit minded, and this is for all nations.

"On this very ground more than a hundred years ago, the four holders of the white buffalo calf woman pipe – from the four corners of the native people's nation - came together in a Sundance ceremony. It was during this ceremony that Sitting Bull had his vision for what was needed to defeat the whites, and protect and preserve his people from the armies that were coming to annihilate them."

The thought of Sitting Bull's prophecy entered my head.

Soldiers falling into the village.

"I am going to pray," Frank said. "Be ready. Because you're going to receive communications from the spirits, and your life will not be the same."

As he chanted in his language, I knelt beside him. Closing my eyes, a flood of colors registered in my brain, the most prominent of which was red.

"Red represents Mother Earth," Frank said. "That's who we are. Our blood is red. We all come from the same place. Black-white-yellow-red - we are a hundred percent related. We come from the Creator."

"I hope that we can find common ground here," he concluded...

CHAPTER ONE HUNDRED AND SIXTEEN

Preparing to leave Frank asked if we could return in January for a commemorative ceremony called the Fort Robinson Breakout Run.

"A hundred years ago many of my people died in that Breakout," he said. "They were fighting for the lives of their children and grandchildren. If it hadn't been for their sacrifice, there probably would be no Northern Cheyenne people."

"So, can you do it?" he asked. "I think you would be a natural for it. I think it's part of your calling. I think you would help the direction we're going. I think you're part of it somehow. You need to come back and sweat."

I would love that, I responded.

He stepped back as though unsure what I'd said.

"Well, we love you, too," he said...

Driving along the highway, there were signs to the Little Bighorn Battlefield National Monument. Thinking about our conversations with Frank, I asked April if we could go?

Driving to the Battlefield April agreed recognized landmarks of the route well enough to lead us on a shortcut.

"I came here once before," she said. "When I was working for NMAI [National Museum of the American Indian]."

She smiled and sat back.

"I was born in the wrong century," she said. "Years ago there was a place for me and the way my mind works, and my ability to recognize small details. I would have been the one who located the place where the herbs and berries grew that were needed for medicines and sacred ceremonies. Now, an appreciation for that doesn't really exist..."

Arriving at the Battlefield we drove the serpentine roads, reading from the placards about the different skirmishes between the Seventh Calvary and Lakota and Cheyenne and Arapaho on that fateful day, June 25th 1876. At a random site I got out of the car.

"I can't imagine the fighting that occurred here," I said, surveying the battlefield. "Men killing each other. The fear they must have experienced."

"I could imagine Frank fighting here," April responded.

Yes, I nodded. That I could imagine. Fearlessly taking to a horse – in a hail of bullets – to protect his people. He would do this. He would have done it a hundred years ago. He battles for his people now.

Then, I recalled something Orville said: When I'd asked how it could possibly be that with everything that had befallen his people – the epidemics of smallpox and measles, the laws forbidding them from practicing their traditions – that certain aspects of their ways weren't lost, he'd shook his head and responded, "It's all here."

The native way is not dead, I thought. It's alive in Frank. In Orville. And Somay. It's being imparted into Wesley. The culture, the traditions, the ways of this people are not lost. They're alive and breathing in them every day...

CHAPTER ONE HUNDRED AND SEVENTEEN

The detour to Montana made it so we had to take the Beartooth Highway to enter Yellowstone. Making our way down the switchbacks, April fought her fear of heights to take in the breathtaking views.

Inside the Yellowstone Park April wanted to tour the geysers. Walking on the wood planks above Old Faithful I observed an excited group of tourists collected around and photographing a small herd of buffalo. I stood clear back, remembering well my face-to-face encounter with a buffalo while wading in the White River on the Reservation. Then, to my surprise, one of the tourists pointed in my direction.

"Hey, look," he said. "Here come a couple more."

Turning, I saw two buffalos moving in my direction, not more than twenty feet away. The first bison was a female; the second was a very large, muscular male, with a numerous scars on its flanks, and a partially amputated tail.

I prayed that they would veer off, but they continued heading right towards me. My heart beating out of my chest, I made myself as still as a tree. After they'd passed, a tourist and park ranger approached me.

"That was the biggest buffalo I ever saw," said the tourist. "Even with you standing on the wood planks, that male buffalo's hump still towered at least a foot over your head as he passed. His shoulders must have been six feet off the ground.

"He must have passed within four feet of where you were standing. If you would have reached out, you probably could have grabbed his horn."

"Be glad that you didn't do that," said the ranger. "This is the mating season, and judging by that stump of a tail that bull had, he'd been in some fights. I think if you would have made any sudden moves, you'd probably still be riding his horn somewhere out in the Park…"

CHAPTER ONE HUNDRED AND EIGHTEEN

Do you wander into places where you should not go? If so, heed bear's warning that being unaware of your limits in certain settings can lead to disaster.
~ Gary Buffalo Horn Man and Sherry Firedancer.

Continuing through the Park, we saw a line of cars parked on the side of the road.

"When you see a whole bunch of cars stopped on the side of the road, it usually means there's an animal sighting," April said.

Indeed, a group of tourists were gathered behind some logs in a meadow on the edge of a lake.

"What's going on?" I asked.

"There's a bear and a cub over across the lake," a tourist said.

Removing my binoculars, I followed the movements of the mother bear and her cubs.

"Hey Mike, it's time to head off," April warned. "That bear is heading our way."

I shook my head, too enthralled to leave.

"OK, it's about time to retreat," April reiterated. "Other people are having the same thought. It's time to retreat."

The bear was moving diagonally.

"Mike, the bear is almost across the lake," April said. "I don't feel safe. I'm going back to the car."

Adjusting the eyepieces, I continued to follow the bear.

"Hey, Mike, I'm out of here. I think you should come with me. Everyone else is gone."

But I stayed, watching the mother bear and her cub, till I found that no matter how I adjusted the eyepiece, the bear remained out of focus?

Looking up from the binoculars, the bear was not more than twenty yards away. That and its diagonal path had nearly cut me off from the car. I looked up at April, who called back to me.

"Mike, play dead," she shouted. "Play dead."

But the thought of lying motionless while a full grown grizzly sat munching on my arm seemed impossible, and I went running to the car. Tumbling into April's arms, she laughed.

"You just have too much animal magnetism," she said...

CHAPTER ONE HUNDRED AND NINETEEN

Leaving Yellowstone we traveled back towards Rapid City, and took a room in Sturgis with a view of Bear Butte. In the wee hours of the morning I awoke to see April standing at the balcony.

"Mike, it's started," she said, pointing outside to the sunrise. "You can just begin to see the outlines of Bear Butte. Come and look. It looks just like a bear - with the stars twinkling all around it."

From the darkness came a blue light that awakened and illuminated the Butte; the saw-tooth pattern of trees below yielded to smooth contours of rock at the higher elevation.

In a few days it was *Yom Kippur* – the Jewish Day of Atonement. Staring at the Butte, the words of the rabbi from last year's *Kol Nidre* service entered my head.

"You bring forth day and night. You transform light into darkness, and darkness into light. There can be no light without darkness. There can be no joy without sadness. No wholeness without brokenness."

Soon this high holy day would begin again, I thought, and I'd be here, and April would again attend these services alone.

Then, looking out at the Butte, instead of a bear, I saw the body of a Native American man resting on a funeral pyre; his chest was muscular, and seemingly raised to the heavens, as though pierced, and instead of the tree of life, tethered to the stars. His arms were well-developed and at his sides; the slope to his abdomen suggested an emaciated form. And gazing at it, I felt sad that here at this sacred site all I seemed to see was death.

Perhaps this is the sacrificial man, I thought. The native sacrifice, like the ceremonies in which they offer their flesh for Mother Earth.

Why do I see such things? Was I thinking about Lyle and what I'm going back to? Is it because I'm concerned that my time on this planet is coming to an end? With no children, when I'm gone, all of me gone, and all I see is death, and nothing left at all.

"These services are really serious," my rabbi had said. "They determine who will be inscribed in the book of life. Who will live, and who will die."

Maybe, you could lay me up there to die, too, I thought. Alone. No one to carry on my name – my line. All gone.

I am that infinite power that drove you out from Egypt. For you were once slaves and strangers there.' May His love never deny us. You are the spark of the divine. And you shall love thy neighbor as yourself. For God is your life and the fullness of your days...

Then, as the sun's rays more illuminated the Butte, the muscular chest of the figure I perceived seemed to glow and radiate, as though pouring huge amounts of energy out into the universe. It was as though this 'muscular' way of living – the traditional way in which native peoples once lived and now honor in their ceremonies – had transformed them somehow? Or was transforming? So to suggest that a life lived this way - in this plane - could in the end put energy into the universe to perhaps help sustain life in another?

"Isn't it in physics that they say that energy is never wasted?" April asked. "Just transformed from one form to another? The ancients seemed to grasp that. They said that in a moment of death, they would see a change. Maybe that's why they performed animal sacrifice at the Temple... I guess they were OK with it because they felt like they owned the animal. It belonged to them. They could do with it what they wanted."

The thought repulsed me, and seemed an unfair and unkind way to treat another being.

"Maybe that's why the Temple was destroyed," she added. "So that animal sacrifice would end, and we could all move beyond animal sacrifice to lives of prayer and service."

Once there was a people, I thought, who lived in harmony with nature; saw themselves not above their fellow creatures, but equal to them. And in their way of life, they captured a way of living and being and thinking and feeling that was truly spiritual – that truly connected them with the Great Spirit. And truly took them to a higher spiritual level than any people I'd ever known.

And looking out again, more than the chest, now the perceived head of the monolithic mountain figure was radiating out energy into the universe, with a yellow light that beamed from its forehead.

April looked around at the other surrounding mountains and buttes.

"None of them seem to be shining that way," she said. "Do you think it's a usual occurrence? All that shining! Like the sun. It's just shining! Maybe that's why this one is holy to the native peoples here?"

Maybe they've made it that way, I thought, through their prayers?

And then the whole figure radiated with light. It was as though to say that life was never wasted. Every life can give rise to some transformative energy that goes out and influences the entire universe. Truly, you save one life, you change the world.

"It would be awesome to do a Vision Quest here," April said.

Yes, maybe I could ask my questions here? Ask what was the right road? Stay and help the native peoples here in the Great Plains? Or, given the opportunity, go to IHS headquarters? Was that the right thing to do?

Then it seemed the Butte were disappearing.

"The light interacts with it in such an unusual way," April said. "It's weird. It's there, but it's like… Shrouded. It's interesting how light literally shrouds it. Till barely a presence remains. If I was writing a poem I'd say, 'The light shrouds it to a partly hidden presence. It's there, but it's not there. Almost like the light is more important than the details.'

"It's like what the sun does to the moon. When the sun hits it, it becomes more about the light that radiates out than the contours of the moon - the skin of it. Like the difference between a regular moon and a blood moon?... A blood moon is what happens when the earth blocks the sun's light on the moon, but you can still see it. The regular moon looks flat and shiny; a blood moon, it's like you're just seeing the outside of it – it's skin. The light is kind of doing something similar to this butte. It becomes more about the light reflecting off of it than the skin of it in that specific moment."

Yes, as though the 'skin' were to keep from our eyes the spiritual being that exists under this covering of flesh. It doesn't matter what you look like – how much money you have, what position you hold. What matters is the person underneath. There's a light under the skin that covers we spiritual beings.

"But it's always changing," she concluded. "It's not like that all the time. Just right now…"

CHAPTER ONE HUNDRED AND TWENTY

Heading to the airport April pointed at a field of sheep, noting that they'd all been recently shaved.

"It's like a concentration camp for sheep," she said.

Yes, I thought. The factory for meat. Using animals as a source of harvest. As if they were plants to be seeded and harvested. How is this respecting one's relations.? Just treating them like dumb animals with no respect. Certainly not like nations the way that the Lakota saw them. Just species to be subjugated. That's what this culture is done. No wonder native peoples can't reconcile with it. It must turn their stomachs.

I was no longer comfortable in it. I had changed. I might as well have been converted. April had joked that I was Jewish because my mother is Jewish, but actually I was a practicing Lakota.

Yes, my eyes have been opened, I thought. I feel for my relations; I feel for the other nations.

"I feel like I'm changing, too," April said...

CHAPTER ONE HUNDRED TWENTY-ONE

At the airport April held me.

"Michael, I'll probably never be able to have children," she said. "It means the end of your line."

"When I first got here, I was kind of amused by some of the names of my patients," I said. "Family names like 'Kills in Water' and 'Crazy Cat.' They'd been translated from Lakota into English. It turned out that most were the names of great chiefs."

"My favorite is 'Makes Room for Them'," I continued. "April, it's OK. Someone else can have my place in line."

She nodded.

"You want to go to the places that it's hard to work," she said. "You want to go and help the people who can't really give you back the things that most doctors want back. And you go to the people who need the most, and you just give them everything, and I really value that. I value what you do. You're amazing.

"And somewhere along the way, I decided to be your support. To make your career, and your job, be what was important. But then, I don't know? Now, you have this job, and your happy here, and people are happy with you, and it feels really stable. And I'm trying to go back to what makes me, me. And in some ways what attracted you to me was to pick that person back up, and build them back up? Does that make any sense to you?"

Her face lost expression.

"I felt totally unprepared for grandma's death," she said. "Didn't know what to do. I wasn't prepared in any way, shape or form. I blamed hospice for it. I was never taught how many drops of morphine to give. I just did it. And I didn't feel supported in anyway by them. I was really mad at them. And I know it wasn't all their fault. I just wound up catching that ball. Because you couldn't have ripped me away from her.

"It's taken me a year now to get over it. I know you know I went into a deep depression, and I was all caught up in it emotionally."

She sighed.

"Before that, when she would start going downhill for some reason, and she was really ill, I would fly out, and be there, and solve what I could. But then I realized that when you get to a place where you can't solve it, that it's not just enough - but a lot - to just hold their hand and walk it with them."

She began to cry.

"You can't solve it in the end," she said, "but you can be there."

She shook her head.

"I was grieving so hard, Mike," she said. "She was more than a grandma for me. She was part mom.

"I was the first grandkid. And my mom was sick. She had some kind of infection. And they couldn't treat her because she was pregnant with me, and it was the last stages of the pregnancy. So they said they were going to wait until I came out, because they had to do some x-rays, and give hard-core antibiotics, and other things. So they waited until I came out. And my mom was in the hospital. And they did some treatments to her. So I was never breast-fed because the tests and treatment meant the milk wasn't healthy for me. So I was taken to my grandmother's, and my grandmother took care of me for a while when I was first born. So my mom thinks my grandma bonded to me, because she had me when I was a newborn. So, she felt very close to me. And I felt very close. Closer than a grandma."

I remembered that last night; when April stayed at her grandmother's side when all other family members had parted; and the light that seem to shine from her the following morning. I wanted to tell her she'd done everything she could. Everything important.

"After she died, I couldn't let go of that," she continued. "I couldn't let go of her. And it took me a long time before I could choose what memories of her I wanted to focus on. Until I could choose to go to when she was a fully adult-capable woman, and concentrate on that. And let go of the sick years."

"If there was a silver lining," she concluded, "it was that she had several years where she was declining. She had stopped being my confidant several years before she died. Probably around three or four. And I had noticed it. And that was the silver lining, because I had to come to terms that I was losing my advisor, I was losing this parent figure. And not only that, I was becoming her care figure, so that our roles were becoming reversed. And I just had to be with her with that. I had to expect that – even though I was grieving the loss of that parent figure. Because for me it was a loss. But she needed me. I couldn't be going over there angry, 'What's happening? You're my parent figure!' I had to be there with her where she was. So I had to go there and change over from being the child to the parent."

Her flight was announced, and a line was forming. I told her I was sorry things turned out the way they did, and it had been such a difficult journey.

"When you say that it's been a terribly difficult journey, much of this has been amazing," she responded. "When I was at NMAI [National Museum of the American Indian], the art and culture was amazing. I was really looking at everything like an artist – really appreciating the visual of things. The creation. The cultural stories that came with them. But never really looking at the condition of the people living it. And you having the experience of basically being embedded the way you have, and sharing with me these amazing people of the Northern Plains – Lakota and Cheyenne – has slowly opened my eyes to the social and human cost to a lot of these cultural things. So that I see them differently. And it gives it a different feel. A real one. It's a little bit like when I was a kid, and I would walk down the street, and would see an oil slick on the road, and I look at it, and think, 'That's really pretty.' You have the different reflections of the colors. And it is pretty. It's like a soap bubble. But now, when I look at it, I go like, 'Oh my God, it's in the water, and it's going to be really bad for everything downriver from here.' So I can see it's pretty, but there is also something really destructive about it. And so I see it more clearly. And I think you've always seen that… I think you have. You've always seen the beauty with also seeing the negative. The destruction. You're more open-eyed then I am on that level. I'm more open-eyed on the personal level of it – 'How is this going to affect me?' But you – You walk into a situation, and not protect yourself. And not think about it at an angle of, 'This is not going to be good news for me.' You just don't look at things that way. The beautiful thing about you is that it makes you want to go in and fix it. Instead of turning away, and not look at it, you look at it, and think, 'How can I fix this?'…"

CHAPTER ONE HUNDRED TWENTY-TWO

Returning to the Reservation, I experienced a sense of reverie; badlands interlaced with growing trees and meadows; buffalo grass blowing in the Plains wind. Arriving at Somay's, Ini was in the yard; opening the gate, she danced all around me, leaping for joy.

Somay wasn't home. I took Ini for a walk along the river. Peering into a thicket of slender trees, I saw a figure resembling Somay; her head bent, she looked like an angel, motionless and silent, as though engaged in prayer. Moving closer, it was a hallowed tree carved by nature. As I stood admiring, I thought it contained Somay's essence. April's, too...

CHAPTER ONE HUNDRED TWENTY-THREE

Returning, Somay still wasn't home.

"We're all at the hospital," she whispered into the phone. "Dad's making ceremony for Lyle."

"Lyle's there?!" I said.

I rushed to the hospital. Climbing the stairs I arrived on the ward just as the ceremony was concluding. From the hallway, I saw Orville in the room; dressed in traditional garb, he stood with his eyes directed to the heavens; arms extended; an eagle fan in each hand. In front of him, Lyle lay motionless in bed, his eyes closed.

Dr. Curtiz was standing nearby. The smell of sage filled the room, and, looking up, I was surprised to find the smoke detectors covered.

"What's going on?" I whispered to Curtiz.

He closed his eyes and nodded, then pulled me aside.

"In their tradition, when a spirit leaves the circle, smoke is used to carry grief away," Curtiz said. "This is a hospital meant to serve native people. The way I see it, if a native patient wants a ceremony, I'm not going to stand in the way..."

Returning to the room, Orville was quietly putting away his pipe, eyes directed downward. Kneeling beside Lyle, I felt for a pulse. He was gone...

"Neither way was wrong," April said. "You lean towards the rules; Dr. Curtiz doesn't lean by them as much, and was comfortable with them having the ceremony. You didn't want to take responsibility for doing something that you didn't feel was totally safe. And that's a reasonable point. I mean, I can understand both of those."

But I felt terrible.

What does it say of me? I thought. That I would say 'No' to a native patient's request to perform a tradition ceremony, while another provider would tell them 'Yes'?

"It's not your fault," she said. "You were just being concerned for everyone in the hospital, instead of just one patient."

"Really, this should have never happened," she added. "If it was so important for native patients to be able to perform their ceremonies, the hospital should have been equipped with a special room for that, instead of doctors scurrying around the rules…"

CHAPTER ONE HUNDRED TWENTY-FOUR

I didn't request leave to attend Lyle's wake and funeral.

"Will Dr. Curtiz be going?" April asked. "If not, I think he would appreciate if you did. If you were one of those doctors who was only there for three months, then – hell, no – you should be at the clinic doing your work. But seeing that you've been there for a while and they're hoping you're going to stay, I think it would probably mean a lot to the community if you went to the funeral..."

But I couldn't. I felt I'd betrayed Lyle – betrayed Orville, betrayed the Tribe – by not honoring their wish to have a ceremony in the hospital, and causing him to leave, and no doubt suffer.

It was Yom Kippur, and I spent the day fasting.

"We come to repent our sins," I recalled our rabbi telling the congregation. "There's nothing more beautiful than to ask for forgiveness. There's not a single one of us who has not missed the mark. Most important is to ask for forgiveness."

Checking the mail, there was a letter from IHS Headquarters.

Congratulations, this letter confirms your selection as Deputy Director, Office of Clinical and Preventive Services in Rockville, Maryland...

CHAPTER ONE HUNDRED TWENTY-FIVE

As I sat re-reading the letter, a knock came from the door.

"How's it going, Doc?" Ryan asked. "We didn't see you at the wake. Orville and Somay were asking about you. I just thought I better come over and make sure you were alright."

I confided my reasons for not attending.

"You didn't fail anyone, Doc," he said. "You were just doing what you thought was right."

Anyway, I said, I was accepted for a position at IHS Headquarters, and would likely be leaving soon.

He depressed the corners of his lips.

"Is that in Washington, DC?" he asked. "The Tribal President asked me one time to go to Washington with a delegation from the Tribe. We got there and this one Senator on the Committee of Indian Affairs - says to me, 'You Indians back again looking for handouts?' I just put me head down and didn't say anything. To guys like him, what happens on the Reservation doesn't matter - because they don't have to live it. But it does matter – because we do live it.

"They have one perception - that Native Americans are all drunks. And the kids are mistreated. So, they say, 'Oh, yeah, we're going to come in with this new educational program. We're going to give them breakfast in the morning.' They'd come to the Reservation, and pick a family, and say, 'Oh, we're doing this on the Reservation. We're doing that.' And they gave this family new clothes and got them all spiffed up for pictures. They fixed their house. And then, they left; and within a year, it was like none of it ever happened.

"It's all about all this hoopla – So they can say, 'We started this new program. We're feeding kids fruits and vegetables in the morning. We're going to educate them about the food tree and everything like that.' So it's like they want to do all the fluff, but they don't want to hear about the real problems.

"I've seen the worst of the Reservation, and I've seen the best of it. What the government said it would provide, and what it didn't."

He shook his head.

"When you go to Headquarters, you should never withhold the truth," he continued. "As a Native American, I would rather you tell the truth of what happens here, then not tell the truth. Because I would trust you more if you would tell the truth, then if you wouldn't tell the truth.

"Because how are you going to educate the people? How are you going to educate anyone? If they just have a certain perception of how it is, rather than the full picture?

"Because the real thing we don't like are people who have a certain perception of the Reservation. That we're moneygrubbing, cheese loving, government welfare…"

He broke off.

"And we're not that. It's what the government made us. They made us reliant on them. We were totally self-reliant. Doing our own hunting, fishing. Doing everything for ourselves. Then, all of a sudden, they had outposts throughout the Midwest, and then the Plains, and they're saying, 'Hey, during the winter, why do you have to go hunt? Why do you need to go and do this? Why do you need to go do that? We'll give you food. We'll give you blankets. We'll give you liquor. Just come to us. Just rely on us. You don't need to go out there and hunt. You don't need to be an Indian.' Then, once we got hooked on that, they put us on Reservations. That's where I think the welfare system came from. We weren't bothering anyone. We weren't raping the land."

He looked out.

"So, now you have huge cattle ranches everywhere. Here, and in Colorado, and in Utah."

He shook his head.

"Yeah, we have our drug addicts. We have our drunks. But what society doesn't? You want to pick at us – but being a sovereign nation, show me the people that don't have the same problems living outside the reservation.

"And, in general, we take care of crimes a lot better than they do on the outside. You commit a crime out there, they want to arrest you, prosecute you, and throw you in prison. On the Reservation, it isn't like that. Because on the Reservation, we're all family. Even if you aren't a straight descendent, we're all family. We got the criminal type. We've got drug addicts. We got people making meth on the

Reservation. There's all that. And they do get prosecuted. But if you see somebody walking down the road, even if they're drunk, my first reaction is to take care of them. My first thought is, 'Let me take him home.' Or let me go take him to where I know he lives. Do something. On the outside, you drive down the road, you see somebody who's drunk or needs help – and you're afraid to help them! Because you don't know how that person's going to react. Are they going to say you rob them? I mean, that scares me. It literally scares me. On the reservation, I can go and even if I don't know them, and I see they're drunk, I can say who my family is, and it will calm them down because all of our families are known, and then I can take them home. On the outside, in the city, I'd be afraid of being mugged.

"So I'd rather have somebody tell the truth about how it is. So that people understand – rather than to sugarcoat it and say, 'I really don't want to say how it is.' I'd rather have somebody educate about how it is, then to have somebody 'uneducate' about it, and then have new docs step on the Reservation and say, 'What the hell?! I didn't know that was there!' That's why I asked you what was your reaction when you first came to the Rez? Because we get people who have never seen the Rez..."

CHAPTER ONE HUNDRED TWENTY-SIX

Sitting alone after Ryan departed, I thought of Orville, feeling sad that I certainly must have disappointed him over the passing weeks.

"I think Orville is a really good man," April said. "His experience reminds me of my grandmother's. You know she was the only member of her family to survive the Holocaust, then essentially devoted her entire life to helping children as a social worker. They were both exposed to malevolent acts that took them away from the entire world that they grew up in – their childhood homes. And instead of becoming hateful and cynical, they chose to reach out and embrace life. Grandma with needy kids and their families, and Orville reaching out to everybody with his culture – and still being inclusive."

"This culture destroyed his culture," she continued, "and still he reaches out to people like you, and shares his culture. What kind of strength, what kind of love, makes it so a person can do that? Instead of being angry and bitter, and wanting to use that against you?"

"It took that terrible year at FQHC for you to go back there," she concluded. "Stan was gone, but Orville stepped up and opened his home and family to you. You've been totally blessed with the deep relationships you've had with the people there…"

CHAPTER ONE HUNDRED TWENTY-SEVEN

Orville led the funeral procession; a rider-less horse representing Lyle on this day; the caravan stretching what seemed like a mile, and everywhere people on the road were holding signs, waving flags, and there were even drum circles.

"Lyle was a respected war veteran," Somay said. "He was wounded in the Korean War and then was released and went back to battle after nineteen days. He was then captured by the Chinese. He was with other Lakota soldiers, and they figured out how to escape. By that time Lyle had gangrene in his stomach, and knew he couldn't make the journey. He sang his fellow warriors the Lakota Flag Song and they were able to make their escape. Lyle was listed as POW/MIA for the next two years until the war ended. When he returned, he was treated like a hero."

Looking out, it seemed he was still respected as a hero, the route lined with proud Lakota people, saying goodbye.

"Lyle's spirit will travel for four days," Orville said, "then enter the happy hunting grounds, to see all the Chiefs, and all of the families, and all the relations that went to there before him.

"It is our tradition, it is our way that when a spirit leaves our circle we use smoke to carry our grief away. You know, when we lose a loved one, we never forget. We never do. We always remember, even when they are in the spirit world. And when we remember, it is always in a good way. We remember the good times, and don't cry for them to come back. Because if we do, they do come back, and they have to suffer just like we are, and we want them to be happy..."

Near the casket were a number of neatly arranged photos of Lyle from different times in his life. Looking at them I was struck by the difference in his appearance when I compared photos from his youth (in which he appeared anxious and afraid) to those later in life.

Lyle He Shields Them was born March 2, 1938, the memorial read. He grew up in Spring Creek. He served in the U.S. Army in Korea...

"He had it really tough as child," Somay said. "Terrible childhood. He went between foster homes, until he finally ran away and joined the Army."

He worked at the elementary school, first as a janitor and later as a bus driver. Lyle enjoyed his job there and was well liked by the students and staff alike...

"When he returned, the tribe really took him in. He was a Sundancer all the way through. The community meant everything to him. Yes, it was there that he was really happy."

Mementos from Sundance ceremonies stretched across the table.

"The Sundance grounds were his favorite place," Somay continued. "Dad told Lyle he could be buried there, and Lyle said he'd liked that."

May he rest in Peace.

"Lyle told me you weren't what he expected," she said. "He was expecting you to be gruff... For you to come in and give him just a few minutes of your time and then walk out again. Instead, what he got was compassion and respect. He said he totally felt comfortable talking with you and telling you the truth..."

CHAPTER ONE HUNDRED TWENTY-EIGHT

After the funeral service Orville called me over.

"Com'on, Doc," he said. "We're having buffalo stew."

Feasting on stew and fry bread, I sat thinking about the weeks I'd cared for Lyle and my experiences, in general, on the Rez. So much had happened. It'd been less than two years, yet it felt like a lifetime.

Ryan came and sat next to me.

"I hope I didn't offend you with what I had to say yesterday," he said. "I was just telling you things from my point of view."

We talked more about the Headquarters position and what I hoped to achieve there, like promoting the 'love and work' concept, and attempting to facilitate employment.

"Awesome," he said. "I'm not sure how entrenched the 'entitlement' or 'hang around the fort' element has become among many of our relatives. I have witnessed mismanagement and poor work ethic again and again on the Reservation. People are more skilled at attracting such opportunities to the Reservation than they are in sustaining and growing them. But I love the idea, and were I a young man, I'd either immerse myself in building work/business infrastructure, political infrastructure or both."

I nodded, though, still, I was not fully certain about the answer to that issue; I feel that respect for the nature on the Reservations is part of the process of restoring that spirit. The years that I'd spent on the Reservation felt like living in a pristine national forest; I thoroughly enjoyed my time taking hikes on the Eagle Trail and wading in the White River; having attended numerous Sundance, Sweat Lodge, Wiping-Away-the-Tears and other ceremonies here, I felt a reverence for the land went hand-in-hand with preserving

Lakota traditions, and it would be my sincere desire that any ventures in employment work closely with the tribe, to see that the nature is honored, and traditional ways preserved.

"That's pretty good to hear," Ryan said. "Because we tell people, 'It's way different than the outside.' But you have to see the beauty - just like when you move to any different town. It could be crime ridden, but you have to see the beauty that's within it. Sure, this happened and that happened, but you have to go out into the nature.

"When I leave and then go back to the reservation, I don't care what happened. The night before there could've been a shooting, or someone injured. I just enjoy the beauty. I enjoy the nature. I go out into the mountains and enjoy the fishing, looking out and seeing the river and buttes or whatever else..."

CHAPTER ONE HUNDRED TWENTY-NINE

Taking a break in my moving preparations I went to the
fairgrounds for the annual Pow Wow. In time with the drum circles,
Lakota dancers performed a myriad of traditional dances. Some wore
regalia made from buckskin and feathers, while others wore bright
colors and exhibited dazzling moves. Orville was on the podium,
serving his usual role as MC.

"Do you dance, Dr. Mike?" Orville asked.

I told him I had performed in an Israeli Dance Troupe.

"Then, you should dance in the intertribal," he said. "That's
when everyone is invited to go out and dance in the circle. You
should go and represent your tribe."

Having always been moved by the Lakota drums and chanting
from the first, I required little incentive to join in. Making my way
between the dancers, I thought at times I chose the wrong direction,
following a shawl dancer moving clockwise in the circle when it
seemed the young men were going the other way. Still, most smiled,
and there was not a disparaging expression among them. Afterwards,
Orville motioned me to the podium.

"I think you would make a good grass dancer, Doctor," Orville
said. "My daughter could make a grass dance regalia for you. She
used to do that for my son."

He sat back.

"Up until when I was sixteen, I used to dance. I was a traditional
dancer. When I was in that boarding school and my mom died, I
didn't dance because I didn't have the regalia. My son was about
three years old and we went to a gathering in Parmalee. We were
sitting there and the announcer says, 'There's a dancer here. And this
family has this bustle especially made out of eagle feathers for a

245

child. There's a dancer in here. And they want to give this to him.' And they called out for my son. So we went out and here was this beautiful eagle bustle for a child. Beautiful!

"But he was only three years old, so we hung it up. When he would ask about it, I would tell him what it is. Then, when he was about four or five years old, he said, 'Dad, I want to dance at the fair.' So I went around and got the other stuff for him. Headpiece. Bells. I got him all set up. And before the fair, I dressed him to make sure he had everything. He stood there looking at himself. Then, he looked at me and said, 'Dad, I want you to dance with me.' And I didn't have anything. Not even one feather.

"I said, 'I don't know. I don't know where to get the regalia.' And here a friend of mine was sitting nearby, and he said, 'I have an extra set. You can use it.'

"So that fair, we dressed up, and some of those old-timers really looked at me, and came over, and said, 'Welcome back.' And as soon as we went into that Grand Entry - as soon as that music started - I was home. It felt so good to dance. Because I knew the songs.

"And afterwards, an elderly woman from St. Francis announced that she was glad to see me back in the center, and donated on my behalf. I never felt so welcome.

"So my son really brought me back to dancing. And he became a champion dancer. He won all over the country. He and Somay would take off and hit the powwow Trail, and did good.

"These are things that we have. They're little things. But it tells you who you are."

Listening, I nodded.

How could I leave? I thought. Orville has cancer. Very soon, he might need my help the way Lyle did.

"Did I tell you we were invited to perform in Italy – my son and me?" he said. "Yeah, dancing. So we were traveling the country performing there, and then my son says, 'Dad, I've been talking to these people at the monastery, and they say that if I want to, I can stay. I feel like I need to be exposed to a different way.' I said OK, and he spent a few months there. When he came back, he said, 'Dad, we'd go out and offer assistance, without asking for anything in return. We'd go and we'd help. Wherever it was, it didn't matter. Every day. And if someone offered us something to eat, then we ate. But if no one gives us anything through the day, then we didn't eat.'

"The time for him that he stayed at that monastery, it had such a profound effect on my son – on his outlook on life. When he got to see it from a different view. And it helped him understand our culture better. 'It's all there in our Sundance and our ceremonies,' he said.

"He was fortunate to have that opportunity. But most of us here don't have that, so we listen, and we hear. Maybe something inside you will click, like it did for my son. But it's kind of hard..."

CHAPTER ONE HUNDRED THIRTY

Passing a drum circle Somay was teaching a group of tourists a dance. They were holding hands, and Somay was instructing them on foot placement. As the steps appeared familiar (like a 'grapevine' in a Jewish circle dance), I joined in. But as the beat of the drum grew faster, the tourists peeled off from the circle, leaving Somay and I dancing on opposite poles. She turned one way and then the other, and I matched her; her steps were more grounded, whereas mine were as though in flight.

Then, crossing the center of the circle, she approached me. Appearing young and strong, her movements portrayed a certain fierceness, force and strength.

Ultimately, I tired (feeling my hamstrings tighten) and put up a hand. She slowed, and this time I crossed the center. Stopping alongside her, we each kneeled, and I whispered in her ear.

"I'm going to have to hand this round to the warrior woman," I said.

She smiled, shook her head, then bent low and put a hand to grip my ankle.

The drumming stopped and loud whooping cries rang out, as those around the circle applauded...

CHAPTER ONE HUNDRED THIRTY-ONE

Passing Somay's on a walk with Ini, she greeted us holding a letter in her hand.

"I was offered a position with the University here," she said. "Their professor of Ceramics left, and the position came open. They asked me to teach…"

As we walked into the Plains together, I confided my concern for her father.

"Dr. Mike, there's no need to feel guilty," she said. "I know you're on the verge of making a big career move, and having second thoughts with all the uncertainty and second guessing it entails. 'Will you be able to correct what feel are imbalances in medicine? Was applying for this position a mistake? Or is it what you were meant to do?' You don't know. You are clear about your values and how you wish to work and live, but you aren't clear about who you are and what you should really do at this juncture. Low hanging familiar fruit is always attractive – Wesley, dad, me. But the universe has presented you with a new opportunity – You've got a place at IHS Headquarters now. It may turn out to be a critical stepping stone, as opposed to a mistake. No matter what direction you ultimately choose, 'doing time' in DC is rarely a bad thing in the long run. Others might not share your dream – so be it. They're not keeping your dream. Whatever dream they're keeping, who knows? But we need people with *Waon'sila* – with compassion."

I nodded. If I could change things for the people here, I had to try. I have loved living in this pristine natural place, but felt the need to try to make things better in a position to do more.

"Maybe you can re-create your life here," she said.

I shook my head. No, I'm going back to all the things there weren't on the Rez. Israeli dancing, karaoke, a nearby airport, malls, temples, Jewish celebrations and all the other non-stop activities I haven't had on the Reservation. I have loved my life here, but I'd only lived it because I had to and wouldn't have that life there.

"So actually when your freedom was taken away," she said, "you found some peace…"

Ini ran ahead. Watching her, I couldn't help but feel a shared pride and admiration.

Not bad for a dog who hadn't had a leg to stand on, I thought. You and me.

She sacrificed herself for you… Maybe, because you're hurting over something and don't even know it. Have a deep wound somewhere that she was sent to heal.

Orville was right. I'd come here a broken creature. As thoroughly broken as Ini's leg. Serving native peoples I'd recovered my dignity. The IHS had given me back my dignity.

Then, it occurred me: Who would keep Ini? I couldn't imagine her leaving this place. How would she take to being in the city on a leash all the time? Where would she roam free?

"Could you really leave without her?" Somay asked. "That dog is the best thing that ever happened to you. Don't you think so?"

Ini sniffed among the buffalo grass and willow trees, before becoming focused on something ahead and initiating slow, deliberate, stealthy steps.

"Look there," Somay said.

In the direction she pointed was an active prairie dog mound. Several of the prairie dogs had strayed a considerable distance from the mound and were in vulnerable positions, and Ini took off like a shot in their direction.

"No, no, no!" I cried. "Don't hurt those creatures!"

Though Ini could have easily intercepted the prairie dogs, she instead immediately stopped on my command, and as the prairie dogs ambled back to their mound, I stood in stunned disbelief.

"You see," Somay said. "She'll listen to you."

Ini again ran ahead – this time disappearing above a ridge. Shortly after, came the sound of barking, and scaling the ridge, Somay and I found Ini on the edge of the woods standing next to a fawn!

"They're the same colors," Somay commented. "The same size. They actually look similar, even though they're different species."

Yes, I thought. Though the fawn was slightly taller than Ini, they were probably the same weight.

"Ini kind of looks like a deer," Somay added. "Maybe the fawn thinks Ini is another deer?"

Noticing Somay and me, the fawn sprang from the open field into the adjacent woods. Ini gave a look as though to say, 'Did you see?!' then leapt into the woods after it, and the two scampered about the brush, jumping and prancing.

Somay laughed.

"They're running around in circles," she said. "Like a couple of little kids."

Ini came out of the woods; but the fawn followed her, as though inviting Ini back to play, and the two jumped back into the woods and frolicked.

"It's like she's saying, 'I like my friend,'" Somay continued. "'It's so much fun to play with my friend...'"

Nodding, I looked on.

Ini finally gets her deer, I thought.

I couldn't imagine seeing anything sweeter...

Making our way back to the house, two more deer appeared on the trail; but this time, Ini made no attempt to run after them and stayed by our side.

"Maybe, it's a sign," Somay said. "She's done what she wanted here and she's ready for something new..."

ABOUT THE AUTHOR

Michael Yanuck MD PhD is a physician-scientist
whose groundbreaking research at the National Institutes of
Health was the basis for a FDA-approved vaccine for cancer.
Following a traumatic leg injury he returned to medicine. Intent on
helping those most in need, he enlisted in the National Health
Service Corps, worked in urban and rural health centers throughout
the country, then served native peoples in the Indian Health Service.
After three years in the field, he was selected Deputy Director of the
Office of Clinical & Preventive Services at IHS Headquarters.

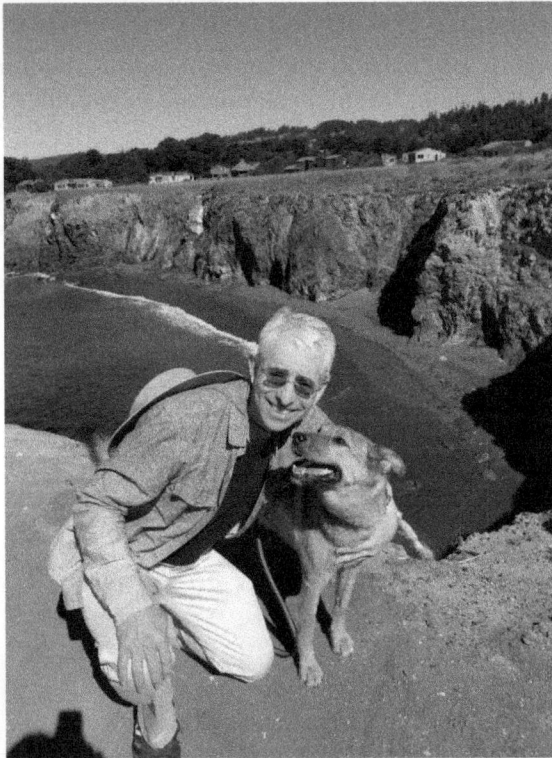

* 9 7 8 0 9 7 4 0 4 5 7 4 0 *